Super Healing

The Clinically Proven Plan to
MAXIMIZE RECOVERY
FROM ILLNESS OR INJURY

JULIE K. SILVER, MD

Assistant Professor of Physical Medicine and Rehabilitation,
HARVARD MEDICAL SCHOOL

RODALE

© 2007 by Julie K. Silver

Rodale books may be purchased for business or promotional use or for special sales. For information, please write to:
Special Markets Department, Rodale Inc.,
733 Third Avenue, New York, NY 10017

Printed in the United States of America

Rodale Inc. makes every effort to use acid-free ⊗, recycled paper ♻.

Book design by Christina Gaugler

Library of Congress Cataloging-in-Publication Data

Silver, J. K. (Julie K.), date
    Super healing : the clinically proven plan to maximize recovery from illness or injury / Julie K. Silver.
        p.   cm.
    Includes index.
    ISBN-13 978–1–59486–631–9 hardcover
    ISBN-10 1–59486-631-7 hardcover
    1. Medical rehabilitation.   2. Medicine, Physical.   3. Healing.   I. Title.
RM930.S55 2007
617'.03—dc22   2007027726

Distributed to the trade by Holtzbrinck Publishers

2   4   6   8   10   9   7   5   3   1   hardcover

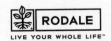

We inspire and enable people to improve their lives and the world around them

For more of our products visit **rodalestore.com** or call 800-848-4735

To my husband and children,
who traveled with me through the Healing Zone
and whose love and support helped me to Super Heal

Contents

Part 3 Fine-Tuning Your Super Healing Plan

Acknowledgments

I very much appreciate the opportunity to share what I know about physical healing with readers. The people who made this possible include my literary agent, Linda Konner, and the acquisitions editor at Rodale, Mariska Van Aalst. Both of these women believed in this book and were instrumental in bringing it to publication. I am deeply grateful for their efforts.

My editor at Rodale, Susan Berg, greatly assisted in making this a better book. She had terrific insights and suggestions, and I incorporated them all. I also want to thank the other publishing professionals at Rodale who worked on *Super Healing,* especially Hope Clarke, Rachelle Vander Schaaf, and Christina Gaugler.

Mary Alice Hanford was terrific about helping me with research and manuscript preparation. Anna Rubin assisted with the Remarkable Recovery interviews. Joel Stein, who is the chief medical officer at Spaulding Rehabilitation Hospital, and Judith Waterston, who is the president of the hospital, have continuously supported my academic work.

I also want to thank Lynn Forde, Stephanie Machell, Alice Richer, and Terry Sutherland for generously offering their expertise. Christine Fennelly, Terry O'Brien, and Alison Bozzi Zaya assisted as well.

As you read *Super Healing,* you'll see that I quoted many people whose words and insights make this a much better book. I am grateful to all of them for their contributions.

Throughout my career, I have had the privilege of watching many incredible people who have faced serious illnesses and injuries. Due to physician-patient confidentiality, I am not allowed to discuss these stories. However, in writing this book, I contacted a number of people who agreed to waive their privacy and share their stories with you. Their courage and kindness in allowing me to tell you about their Remarkable Recoveries is just part of what makes them so wonderful. I hope that you will enjoy their stories and that they will inspire you as you work to heal.

Finally, I am indescribably grateful to my family, friends, and colleagues who have supported me throughout my illness and recovery. All of the things you have done, big and small, made my journey through the Healing Zone more tolerable. I'm sure that your love and support contributed to my ability to heal well.

Introduction

Illness and injury are facts of life. We all get colds and sustain minor bumps and bruises. We expect this and accept it. What is harder to accept is serious illness or injury. Yet this, too, is an inevitable part of most people's lives.

If you are reading this book, there is a good chance that you have had a life-altering medical condition. The good news is that while serious health problems are a normal part of living, your body will work hard to heal whatever is wrong with it. If you have a plan to help your body recover, it is easier to heal optimally. That is what this book is about—how you can help your body to heal as well as possible.

I was diagnosed with breast cancer in my thirties. I certainly wasn't expecting to encounter a life-threatening illness until I was much older. But I also knew from past personal and professional experience that our destinies include facing unexpected and unwanted health crises. Let me tell you about my first.

At age 28, I had officially been a doctor for less than a year and was working as a medical intern in a suburban teaching hospital in Massachusetts when I became a patient myself after going into preterm labor with my first child. The doctor assigned to my case, who never once examined me, instructed the nurse to give me tranquilizers whenever I complained that I couldn't breathe. I can only assume that he thought I was overly anxious and perhaps a bit hysterical about being in labor 2 months before my due date.

As a friend of mine, a fellow physician in training, read the results of my tests, he told me that my blood oxygen level was dangerously low and that my heart was showing serious signs of strain—the sort of strain that appears in the EKGs of people who are having heart attacks. He called for an ambulance and had me transferred immediately to one of the Boston hospitals that specialize in high-risk pregnancies, where I was treated in an intensive care unit setting.

It wasn't until well after I was out of the hospital that I realized that doctor assigned to me had never touched me and had given me inappropriate medications that contributed to my going into congestive heart failure. I was definitely not hysterical, and at least some of my anxiety had to do with the very real fact that I was literally suffocating.

Though I had treated many people with serious medical problems, this was the first time that I faced one myself. The late writer Susan Sontag called this entering the "kingdom of the sick." In a vivid description of moving from good health to illness, Sontag wrote:

> Illness is the night-side of life, a more onerous citizenship. Everyone who is born holds dual citizenship, in the kingdom of the well and in the kingdom of the sick. Although we all prefer to use only the good passport, sooner or later each of us is obliged, at least for a spell, to identify ourselves as citizens of that other place.

Though I temporarily entered the kingdom of the sick, what I recall most vividly is being dreadfully frightened for my son, who also entered "that other place" when he was born a few days later—2 months before his due date. He was tiny, weighing just over 3 pounds, and he needed to be hospitalized for about a month, until he reached 4 pounds and could drink without a tube.

Every day I would sit in a rocker and watch my son in his incubator. Another woman—who had given birth to a son the same day and at almost exactly the same weight—rocked with me. Our boys grew slowly, and we could take them out and hold them only periodically. One day it became clear that her son had stopped gaining weight. He had a congenital heart condition that would require surgery. A major heart operation is extremely risky for a baby weighing less than $3\frac{1}{2}$ pounds, but her little guy sailed through the procedure and began to gain weight again.

Through the years, our families have remained friends. Our sons know each other, and both are thriving. Neither boy pays much attention to the fact that he came into the world far too early and had to rely on the profound healing abilities of his body, which were present from birth. Of course, modern medicine played a role, too. Here is what could have happened if these boys had been born 100 years earlier.

> Standard medical procedure for premature babies before the twentieth century was to assume they would die. French pediatricians Pierre Budin and Martin Couney designed the first incubators for preemies in the 1890s, but they couldn't get investors or medical acceptance for the idea of using them. To garner both, they began to set up exhibits of "incubator babies" at World's Fairs and even amusement parks. Dr. Couney's work in America included a very popular display at Coney Island that ran for 40 years. . . . More than 8,000 premature babies were saved by the

sideshow exhibits. By the middle of the twentieth century, the results finally shamed obstetrical hospitals into investing in their own incubators.

Our boys, now teenagers, are a testament to how modern medicine and our bodies' natural healing ability can work together to Super Heal. We are born with amazing healing powers, which we retain throughout our lives. Perhaps, as with my son, modern medicine saved your life. However, saving a life is only part of the healing journey. A life can be saved in seconds, minutes, or sometimes days. But recovering from a serious illness or injury usually takes months or even years.

I call this time, when the body still has the capacity to further mend, the Healing Zone. During this period, regardless of how long it lasts, you will have a much better chance of healing optimally if you utilize principles of modern medicine that have been proven to assist with physical recovery. In his book *Journey into Healing*, Deepak Chopra, MD, writes, "The reason why not everyone manages to take the healing process as far as it can go is that we differ drastically in our ability to mobilize it." The Super Healing Plan that I describe in this book is a tool you can use to mobilize the healing process.

Working in the Healing Zone

After my son's birth, I was in the Healing Zone for several weeks, while I physically (and emotionally) recovered. During my recuperation, I moved back to Washington, DC, where I had gone to medical school at Georgetown. I spent the next 3 years finishing my training at the National Rehabilitation Hospital as a physiatrist (pronounced fizz-ee-AH-trist)—that is, a doctor who specializes in rehabilitation medicine.

The medical specialty of physical medicine and rehabilitation (PM&R) started as a response to the tremendous need to help soldiers recover from their injuries. During World War II, there were more than 600,000 injured military personnel returning to the United States. Though MASH (mobile army surgical hospital) units didn't materialize until later, medicine had advanced to the point where we were getting really good at saving lives, but we couldn't do much beyond that. People were left to their own devices to heal. Doctors began to explore the concept of training specialists who knew how to promote physical recovery and would work closely with patients in the Healing Zone, using the latest technology and innovative care. These doctors would be experts at helping people to restore function. Hence, my specialty came into being with the mantra "focus on function."

As a physician who specializes in rehabilitation medicine, I have worked for many years with patients who are in the Healing Zone. I direct the care of people with many different kinds of medical conditions—including but not limited to stroke, traumatic brain injuries, sports injuries, neck and low-back pain, multiple sclerosis, Parkinson's, fibromyalgia, post-polio syndrome, and cancer. I also treat individuals with orthopedic conditions that range from sprained ankles and knees to serious multitrauma injuries from car accidents and physical violence.

Washington, DC—then reputed to be the most dangerous place in the country to live, with hospitals filled with victims of violent crimes—was an excellent training ground for someone in my medical specialty. Though it was heartbreaking to take care of people like Sasha Kondratiuk, who was attacked by a knife-wielding man high on PCP, I learned a lot about what it takes to rehabilitate people who are seriously injured. (Sasha was injured nearly a decade after I had moved from Washington to Boston; though she never was my patient, she spent time both at the hospital where I had trained and at Spaulding.)

Sasha is an amazing young woman, and her story is very powerful. Because of this, she was asked to join a special program called Remarkable Recoveries at Spaulding Rehabilitation Hospital in Boston. In this program, we invite people who have lived through serious injuries and illnesses to share their stories and bring inspiration and hope to others who are currently navigating the Healing Zone. Throughout this book, I'll share many Remarkable Recoveries from people who participate in this program. I'll also tell you about others who are not part of this program but have incredible healing stories.

Sasha was very seriously injured; one of the knife wounds to her back left her paralyzed. Today she is able to walk and is in the process of getting an advanced business degree at Oxford University in the United Kingdom. Her boyfriend, Alex, remained devoted to her throughout her ordeal, and the two recently became engaged to be married. Sasha tells more of her story on page 36.

Living in the Healing Zone

Though I had worked with patients throughout my career who, like Sasha, were in the Healing Zone, except for my relatively brief hospitalization for preterm labor complicated by congestive heart failure, I never lived there. That changed in 2003 when I was diagnosed with breast cancer.

Actually, it had begun a couple of years earlier, while I was nursing my youngest child. I felt a thickness in my left breast and began to worry that something was wrong. I stopped nursing before I really wanted to and went to the doctor. My mammogram looked perfect, but I was still concerned, so I went for a second opinion and more tests. Nothing.

Reassured, I went about my daily life and continued to do my monthly breast exams, but I always felt that my left side was a little different. It wasn't a distinct lump, really—just a thickness that was slightly irregular compared with my right side. I knew that our bodies have many asymmetries and chalked it up to that.

More than 2 years passed; my baby grew to a beautiful 3-year-old girl with glorious brown hair and an infectious laugh. And I still couldn't shake the feeling that something was wrong. I told myself that I was wasting my time going back to the doctor. At age 38, I was not even old enough to get a baseline mammogram (usually women get these when they turn 40), and I had already been given two workups. Still, I was worried, so I went for a third evaluation.

This time the breast surgeon, a serious woman, found the tiniest lump when she examined me. She agreed to repeat the mammogram and ultrasound. We talked about a breast MRI (the latest technology), but I opted for the mammogram first. There were two masses and a lot of new calcifications. *Cancer.*

The great irony with cancer is that at the beginning of treatment, you might feel great, but you know that something terrible is going on inside your body. By the end of treatment, you are physically debilitated, but you feel grateful that treatment was even possible. In her book *Flying Crooked,* Jan Michael describes it this way: "Such a weird disease, creeping through your body without your noticing. First you have lumps, but you feel fine. You're whisked into hospital and they mutilate you, and suddenly, you're not fine at all."

As a cancer patient, I lived in the Healing Zone for more than 2 years. When I had been given my last chemotherapy treatment, my oncologist told me, "Now get on with the rest of your life." This was simultaneously heartening and disheartening. I was delighted to move forward, but I was a physical wreck. It was obvious that despite receiving treatment at one of the best cancer centers in the world, I was not going to get advice on physical healing. My doctor's work was done—he had rid me of my cancer, and, save for the occasional checkup to be sure that it did not reappear, I was on my own.

I pause here to say that I had outstanding care throughout my illness, and that my doctors—all brilliant—worked hard to save my life. As oncologists, though, they didn't have the time or rehabilitation experience to help me optimally heal once I finished treatment.

Many patients turn to self-help books during times of illness, and I was no different. During my recovery, I searched for books that focused on physical healing. I was surprised to find that despite the hundreds of books on cancer, there wasn't a single book devoted to physical healing after chemotherapy and other treatments end. There were plenty of books on emotional healing, but no one had written a book about how to physically heal. In short, no medical doctor had ever written about what I and others in my specialty focus on every day, which is how to bridge the gap between what the body can do to heal without any assistance and what it can do to optimally heal with the help of evidence-based medical advice.

As I was healing myself, I thought about my years of medical training and practice. Faced with my desire to heal quickly and feel physically stronger, I needed to distill an incredible amount of knowledge into some basic healing principles that I could follow. I was too ill to think about, much less implement, all of the various healing methods. Instead, I had to decide: What are the best ways? What are the main healing principles, and how can I achieve them with the least effort? Out of this exercise came my first book, *After Cancer Treatment: Heal Faster, Better, Stronger.*

Writing *After Cancer Treatment* forced me to synthesize the medical practices that guide my care of patients who are recovering from cancer and its treatment. It also prompted me to think about how the same practices really apply for the vast majority of my patients recovering from injury and illness, not just cancer. I took these core principles and shaped them into a practical plan that readers can use to help them physically recover. I relied on the best medical research currently available, along with common sense, intuition, and a lot of experience treating people in the Healing Zone.

In conventional medicine—what we refer to as evidence-based medicine—research is paramount. We rely heavily on the results of studies that show us what works and what doesn't. But the research has many gaps. To fill these voids, doctors utilize common sense, intuition, and experience. These skills are what make up the "art" of medicine. A skilled physician is both a scientist and an artist.

In *Super Healing,* I combine the art and science of medicine into an easy-to-follow plan that will allow you—no matter what kind of health problem you are dealing with—to recover as optimally as possible. It may seem odd to you that one plan can work for many different injuries and illnesses, but it can. I'll explain why and how this works in the first chapter.

Just by reading this book, you are doing a lot to help yourself. I wish for you as smooth and complete a recovery as possible.

PART 1

You *Can* Super Heal

Chapter 1

The Power of Super Healing

I wrote this book with the sole purpose of helping you to optimally heal. Of course, I don't know your personal medical history, and the details of that are important. But I can offer advice on how to create your own plan to recover as well as possible. I base all of my recommendations on scientific studies and my many years of experience in rehabilitation medicine. As you read this book and formulate your own Super Healing Plan, I encourage you to work with your doctor, who has important information about your particular health situation.

It might seem odd that a plan that will work for you will also work for other people. After all, illnesses and injuries vary greatly in many respects. Some are curable, while others are chronic and can't be cured, though they can be managed. The reason that you can tailor the Super Healing Plan to help you heal is that in rehabilitation medicine, we use strategies that are designed to maximize physical health in people with vastly different health experiences.

The Many Faces of Illness

In the introduction, I talked briefly about my diagnosis with cancer. Though medical advances have made cancer a curable condition, the treatment is extremely toxic, and patients tend to feel much worse at the end of treatment than at the beginning. Chronic conditions such as multiple sclerosis have their own imprint.

One of the best descriptions I've read highlighting the differences between a condition that can be cured and one that can be managed comes from a book aptly titled *Limbo*. In it, author A. Manette Ansay describes what it is like to have an injury or illness that can be cured.

> [Curable conditions] follow the Aristotelian model of storytelling, the one you had to memorize in high school, the one to which every work of fiction you discussed got strapped, howling, like a martyr to the rack. Each begins with an inciting incident: a mysterious seizure, a freak accident, an inexplicable symptom. This is followed by rising action: the trip to the emergency room, visits to specialists, moments of doubt and despair. Finally, there is a climax: the surgery or treatment, everything touch and go. If there is a supernatural element to this anecdote, it's likely to appear at this point: a tunnel of light, the voice of God, the appearance of an angel. And at last, comes the denouement: a resolution, a cure, or failing that, a clear prognosis, a lesson learned.

Ansay goes on to describe what it is like to live with a chronic condition, for which there is no known cure.

> But what if your story shapes itself differently? What if there is no climax, no resolution, only the passing days, the paralyzing uncertainty, the gradually dawning sense that, regardless of what happens next, you will never return to the country you have left, to the body you once took for granted? What if things simply happen because they do, and then you pick yourself up or not? What kind of story is that?

Another category of illness, which may overlap with the rest of the categories I describe here, consists of those conditions that are "invisible"— that is, they are not obvious to others. Examples include some types of cancer, fibromyalgia, and recovery from a heart attack. This invisibility can be a blessing and a curse. At times it is a blessing because one can "pass" as normal. At times it can be a curse because people may be less sympathetic to those who are ill when they can't see the problem.

In their book *Living Well with a Hidden Disability,* authors Stacy Taylor and Robert Epstein, PhD, explain why living with an invisible illness has its own challenges.

> While living with any disability is difficult, there are unique challenges when your problems are invisible. Your requests for special needs often evoke skepticism. You may therefore have a harder time asserting yourself and feeling entitled to special help.

Trauma is another category that has some unique characteristics. Trauma, such as that sustained by Sasha Kondratiuk (whom you met in the introduction), can leave people with scars and permanent injuries. Though the trauma itself is not ongoing, the disability from it may be lifelong.

A patient of mine whom I'll call Ron was a senior in high school when he got into what he describes as an "altercation" with some other male teenagers. They knocked him to the ground, where he was kicked and pummeled until he was unconscious. During his hospitalization, he was treated for multiple orthopedic injuries, including bone fractures and a traumatic brain injury. Though today Ron outwardly appears to be a healthy young man, he has lingering problems with memory, concentration, balance, and coordination. He has healed well and optimally but not completely.

Permanent problems are not unusual when someone has experienced serious trauma. Still, Ron is doing remarkably well and continuing to focus on maintaining the best possible health several years after his injury.

Why the Super Healing Plan Will Work for You

If you are ill or injured, your medical condition may fit into one of these general categories. But this doesn't mean that you are exactly like anyone else. Your body and what it needs to heal are unique, which is why you should read this book with a discerning eye about what will work for you. I have tremendous respect for what people tell me about their bodies. You probably have great instincts and insight, and it's best to use these skills along with the advice that I offer.

It's also important to understand that regardless of your injury or illness, your body will work in a predictable way to help you heal. This is why my specialty of physical medicine and rehabilitation (PM&R) covers so many medical conditions. Many specialists concentrate on just one part of the body or one kind of ailment. For example, oncologists treat cancer, cardiologists treat heart conditions, and nephrologists treat kidney problems. By comparison, those of us who are rehabilitation doctors, or physiatrists, are experts in helping people heal from a host of medical conditions.

How is it that we can specialize in rehabilitating people with so many different conditions and still be effective? The answer is simple: Healing principles are similar for many injuries and illnesses. Put another way: While the problems may differ quite a bit, the solutions are much the same.

At this point, you may be thinking something like "Does this mean that you can treat someone with pneumonia the same way you treat someone who has been seriously injured in a car accident?" The answer is no and yes. Of course, the person with pneumonia needs antibiotics that can cure the infection, while the accident victim may need surgery and other treatments to repair broken bones. However, if both of these patients require prolonged hospitalizations that leave them weak and unable to function as they normally do, then both of them will enter the Healing Zone. In the Healing Zone, their treatment to achieve optimal recovery will be similar and involve the same basic tenets of rehabilitation medicine. For example, most people in the Healing Zone should focus on rehabilitative measures that:

- Optimize their immune systems to facilitate healing and avoid infections that may be a complication of an illness or injury
- Encourage the healing of skin, bones, muscles, tendons, and nerves
- Build strength and endurance

Why Rehabilitation Works

You may still be wondering how someone who's very sick can be rehabilitated in a similar manner to someone with a traumatic injury. If you have had a serious illness or injury, a major part of healing involves recovering from the "deconditioning" that occurs because you are less active than usual. The more inactive you are, the more deconditioned your body becomes.

One of the most striking effects of bed rest takes place at the muscular level. Research has shown that people on bed rest lose 1 to 3 percent of their strength *per day* over the first 2 weeks. The total loss can climb as high as 50 percent in those who remain inactive for 3 weeks or more. Marked declines in muscular strength occur even in people who are not on bed rest but become sedentary because of a medical condition.

All of this means that you can lose a great deal of strength simply by being less active than usual. Unfortunately, loss of muscular strength occurs with no effort and progresses extremely quickly. Regaining strength takes considerable effort and progresses much more slowly.

While complete inactivity or reduced activity has profound effects on muscular strength, it also leads to numerous other changes that are occurring at the same time. Here is a short list of what else can happen when someone is ill or injured and not able to move about as much as usual.

- Reduced heart efficiency, resulting in decreased endurance
- Bone loss, which can lead to osteoporosis

- Skin changes that may result in poor wound healing, rashes, and pressure ulcers
- Declines in lean body mass and increases in body fat
- Loss of important minerals, including nitrogen, calcium, phosphorus, sulfur, and potassium
- Impaired glucose tolerance
- Altered circadian rhythm
- Reduced breathing capacity
- Impaired kidney function
- Decreased bowel motility
- Problems with balance and coordination
- Poor sleep

Depending on your particular condition and overall health status, you may experience some or all of these changes. Some you might identify with right away because you've been experiencing them yourself (e.g., poor sleep). Others may be affecting your health more silently (e.g., bone loss).

The important point here is that nearly everyone who is seriously ill or injured becomes deconditioned and must work to regain physical strength and health. Rehabilitation principles focus on what we call *reconditioning*, which is the process of helping you to regain as much of your former health status as possible. Super Healing is a structured plan that can help you to reverse the many adverse effects of serious illness or injury.

Looking at it another way, ask yourself: "Will making my immune system stronger, healing my body more quickly, and improving my physical strength and endurance help me?" If you answer yes, then you are in the rehabilitative phase of healing that I call the Healing Zone. This book will help you accomplish all that and more.

Beginning the Journey

In the forthcoming chapters, I focus on the things that are most important in physical healing. I offer a specific plan that will enable you to heal optimally. Of course, this book does not take the place of your doctor's sage advice. It's not a substitute for the personal medical attention that only your doctor can give you. Rather, you should use it *as a general guideline* in addition to working with your physician to determine the best course of action for your particular case.

As you continue to read, you'll notice that I often use the metaphor of taking a journey through the Healing Zone. Because many people view healing as a journey, I adopted this metaphor to describe how to spend your time in the Healing Zone. In the next chapter, you'll board the "train" that will take you on this trip.

Before we begin, I want to emphasize that every healing journey is different, and though a complete recovery is ideal, it is not always possible. Committing yourself to healing is still incredibly worthwhile and will enhance your life in many ways. So even if you are not able to achieve your previous state of health, the journey is well worth it.

Longtime cancer survivor Wendy Schlessel Harpham, MD, describes reaching your final destination as a "new normal." Often when I speak to groups, I talk about this new normal and explain that while it's important to emotionally adjust to the impact of a serious injury or illness, before you do, try to Super Heal. What I find in my medical practice is that some people accept too much pain, fatigue, and loss of function as their new normal, when in fact they could heal more optimally. I don't want you to accept any more pain or disability than you have to.

In Dr. Harpham's book *Happiness in a Storm,* she writes:

> To heal is to lessen a hurt, repair a branch, and create a sense of completeness. To recover is to regain what's been lost. Ideally, healing will lead to your recovery. Yet, even if complete or partial recovery is not possible, you can still take steps to heal as you face ongoing physical challenges and losses. You may have trouble believing it now, but it is possible to end up even stronger and better than ever in one or more ways.

Of course, you probably want the life that you had before you became ill. It's a normal desire; it would be unusual if you didn't feel this way. But you may be interested to know that many people report having better lives *after* a major life event that involves confronting a serious medical condition. Consider this possibility—in the future, you actually can have a happier and more fulfilling life than you had in the past. I certainly don't want to minimize the tragedy associated with illness and injury, but I do want you to know that many people go on to lead wonderful lives despite needing to confront serious health obstacles.

I also want to stress that in order to heal optimally, you'll need both knowledge and determination. Right now you may be feeling discouraged and overwhelmed. Understandably, you may not be interested in putting time and energy into pursuing a plan that will help you heal. This is normal—especially early on during the crisis phase of illness, when people tend to feel overwhelmed and their thoughts are not as focused as usual.

Even if this is true, keep reading, because you'll fulfill the first criterion for healing optimally: knowledge. Knowing what you need to do truly is half the battle. Start with that, and the rest will be much easier to handle. Winston Churchill may have captured this idea best when he famously said, "When you are going through hell, keep going." To this I'll add, no matter how you feel now, keep reading.

Chapter 2

A Ticket to the Healing Zone

A ll aboard!

This book is your ticket to physical healing. For some, completing the trip will take weeks or months; for others, it will take a lifetime. The duration of the journey is not entirely within your control, so it's best to focus on how it will begin rather than when it will end.

You will need to bring along three intangible items and some key traveling companions. Let's begin with the intangibles.

Attitude Is Everything

The first thing you'll need is the proper attitude. This is separate from your personality and your mood; it is something you can shape and control. When I think of the ideal healing attitude, it reminds me of the famous Serenity Prayer, penned in 1926 by the American religious and social thinker Reinhold Neibuhr.

> God grant me the serenity to accept the things I cannot change;
> Courage to change the things I can;
> And wisdom to know the difference.

You don't need to believe in God or have a religious background to appreciate the message in this prayer. Healing is a process that you can help to shape and encourage but cannot completely control. This goes back to the idea that I discussed in the first chapter about the need for many of us to accept a new normal—but before we do, to try to Super Heal.

Before I faced my own healing challenges, I would marvel at my patients, particularly those who approached healing with what I can only describe as grace. Through my observations, I found that the grace with which people dealt with illness had little to do with their diagnosis, age, gender, or any other discernible and perhaps objective factors.

One young woman whom I treated for forearm tendinitis (essentially, tennis elbow) was despondent for weeks because she had to slightly alter her plans to play tennis on her honeymoon, which would likely have aggravated her injury. She once said to me, "This tendinitis is ruining my whole life!"

At about the same time, another young woman came to my center for rehabilitation after being seriously injured in an accident. She had been standing on the sidewalk in front of a grocery store when an elderly man lost control of his car and ran into her. She ended up with a leg amputation. Despite a normal period of tremendous grief and many hours spent in physical therapy, she carried on with her plans to go to college.

Both of these patients are physically attractive, but the young woman who is most appealing is the one with the amputation. There is an inner beauty about her that is truly indescribable. People are drawn to her warmth and her character. In short, she possesses the grace of someone who healed as well as she could and now has gone on with her life. She is not a tragic heroine but an accomplished woman who has successfully navigated serious adversity. She and many others like her were role models for me as I faced cancer and the toxic treatments necessary to prolong my life.

Shaping Your Attitude

While the proper attitude is important for your healing journey, keep in mind that it is normal to feel more or less discouraged at various times during this process. Realistically, it is impossible to have the "perfect" attitude for recovery. Instead, it is something to aspire to, so you may optimally heal.

Of course, at times you may focus on what you can't change and wonder, "Why is this happening?" You may feel angry, depressed, frustrated, or a combination of many other emotions. All this is normal. The goal here is not to fake it and pretend to have the ideal attitude but, rather, to genuinely try to accept what you can't change and instead focus your attention on how you can help yourself heal.

You may be thinking, "How can I accept what has happened to me?" A life altered by illness or injury likely was not in your plans. Claudia Osborn, MD, is a doctor who was hit by a car while cycling. In her memoir, *Over My Head,* she writes about her incomplete recovery from the traumatic brain injury she sustained. In the following passage, she describes what many of us initially feel about our conditions.

One word, hiding in my unconscious, lying in wait on the periphery of my knowledge, had stripped me of hope and shattered my dreams. *Permanent.* How could I continue to live with this deficient brain, continue to exist in the unrecognizable, undesirable being? My head injury was bearable only because it was temporary. Permanent injury meant I had already lost. My job. My identity. My life. I was not this damaged shell of a person. I couldn't be. I remembered and loved the person I was. That was the real me.

It is normal to grieve over what you have lost and worry about what the future holds for you and your family. I encourage my patients to grieve—but I also tell them that they can turn their anxiety to their advantage. For example, perhaps being worried was what prompted you to read this book. Maybe the angst you feel helps you remember to take your medicine every day.

Worry and Acceptance

Worry is closely aligned with uncertainty, and uncertainty is practically synonymous with illness. No one with a health issue is free from the worry associated with uncertainty. While it is true that much of what we count on day to day actually is uncertain, illness takes this unpredictability to a higher level and doesn't allow for even the illusion of knowing what the future holds.

But uncertainty and the worry associated with it needn't rule your life. No one has the recipe for how to live a certain life. We can make plans, and we will realize many of those plans—but not all of them. Instead, the antidote to uncertainty is to minimize how much you let it haunt you in your daily routine. In her aptly titled book *Embracing Uncertainty,* Susan Jeffers writes, "Nowhere has it been proven that a rich, joyous, abundant life cannot exist in the presence of uncertainty." Jeffers suggests that people train themselves to become adventurers rather than worriers.

Worry, in its extreme form, is a diagnosable anxiety disorder. (I'll go into more detail about how mood affects healing later in this book.) But there is one word that can help control your worry or anxiety, and that is *acceptance.* Acceptance is the key to moving down an optimal healing path. When I talk about acceptance, I do not mean that you must approve of or in any way be thankful for this unwanted adversity. Rather, what I mean is that you should focus your attention firmly on those things over which you have some control.

David Leone knows a lot about acceptance. He had recently celebrated his 30th birthday, and he and his wife were anticipating the birth of their first child, when his life suddenly changed due to a serious injury. In his own words, he describes what happened.

> On September 4, 2004, my wife, Michele, and I awoke to a perfect, sunny day. It was Labor Day weekend, and we had plans for a busy 3 days of work on the house. Keeping with our routine, Michele and I started the day with a walk around the neighborhood. Upon returning home, I took the steps that would change my life forever.
>
> We were painting our house, and earlier in the week I had noticed several loose boards against the roofline. With a hammer in one hand and a mouthful of nails, I climbed a ladder to fix them. What I didn't know was that a colony of bees had taken up residence behind the boards. It took only a few blows of the hammer before I found out the hard way. The bees swarmed my face, and before I knew what I was doing, I stepped back off the ladder.
>
> I remember being in midair, and I'm still haunted by that image. I remember wondering if this is how my life would end. The next thing I remember is waking up on the ground, unable to move my legs. What happened next was a blur of images: a neighbor who heard my screams; the look of terror on my wife's face; firefighters; EMTs; police; an ambulance; Medflight. At the hospital, I was told that I had broken my back and crushed my spinal cord. Without significant medical advances, I would never walk again.
>
> A week later I was transferred to Spaulding Rehabilitation Hospital. Within minutes, I met Dr. Kevin O'Connor, who would guide my recovery for the next 7 weeks. Dr. O'Connor set the tone for my therapy. "Consider rehab like a buffet," he said. "You don't have to put everything on your plate right away. Take a little at a time and come back for the rest later."
>
> Toward the end of my stay at Spaulding, I watched a paraplegic peer counselor roll into the building with his 11-month-old son riding in his lap. His son knew no other father than one in a chair and couldn't care less. "That's what I want," I thought. "That's how I want to be with my child."

David's story is compelling; he is a survivor of a serious and life-altering injury. Yet his life is full, with a devoted wife, a new baby, and an exciting career. Though undoubtedly it was incredibly painful, one of the first things David had to accept was that at this time there is no cure for paralysis.

Perhaps one day it will be an option, but for the time being, walking is out of the question. In order to heal optimally, David had to face this hard truth and accept what he could not change.

No matter how you feel about things now, you can shape your attitude into one that will help you heal. Nazi death camp survivor Viktor Frankl reminded us, "Everything can be taken away from a man but one thing: the last of the human freedoms—to choose one's attitude in any given set of circumstances." Thus, the first intangible to pack on your healing journey is an attitude that allows for accepting what you cannot change and working on realistic goals for recovery.

Your Plan of Action

The second intangible is an action plan. Actually, you can turn this into a tangible by writing down your goals. In the next chapter, I will explain how to design healing goals and implement them. At this juncture, let me just say that it is easy to over- or underestimate what you'll be able to accomplish in terms of physical healing.

In August 2001, my uncle—who was then the Olympic sports editor for *USA Today*—called me at home and asked if I would be willing to review the x-rays of two-time Olympic and world champion Hermann Maier, then the most recognizable alpine skier in the world. Maier had been thrown from his motorcycle into a ditch after colliding with a car in front of him. He was airlifted to a hospital in Salzburg, where surgeons spent 7 hours trying to save his right leg. Following the surgery, his kidneys were failing, and there still was a possibility that his leg would need to be amputated.

After hearing about the accident—in which "the Herminator" had sustained nerve damage in both of his legs—and looking at the x-rays of his right leg fractures (both bones in the lower leg had been crushed), I thought that this likely was a career-ending injury for the skiing legend. I gave a quote for the article: "The major concern is infection and will be for quite a while." I also mentioned that while the bones would heal fairly quickly, other more disabling injuries might be problematic (e.g., permanent nerve damage to his legs).

After doing this interview, I didn't think much more about Maier until a short 4 months later, when I read that he was back on skis. At the time, he needed to wear a special boot to protect his right shin, where skin from his left upper arm had been grafted. To my amazement, just 17 months after his truly horrific accident, Maier won a World Cup super-G in Kitzbuhel, Austria.

Few people would have predicted Maier's incredible recovery, yet his story is not unique. You probably have heard about cyclist Lance Armstrong, the seven-time winner of the Tour de France, who endured a difficult physical recovery from advanced testicular cancer that had spread to his brain. These stories made international news, but there are many others from average people who have achieved their own impressive physical recoveries.

Perspective

The third intangible is your ability to weather setbacks. This has a lot to do with perspective. Although you strive to get to your destination as quickly as possible, there may be unwanted stops or detours along the way. Healing almost never occurs linearly, without any dips in the graph. Instead, it often seems like a "two steps forward, one step back" process—or even two steps forward and then a halt, with no further forward or backward movement for a while.

Just knowing that you will almost certainly experience plateaus or setbacks can go a long way in helping you prepare for and overcome them. Later in this book, I'll talk more about how to handle these temporary detours in the healing process.

Your Traveling Companions

Along with the three intangibles—a proper attitude, an action plan, and an ability to weather setbacks—you'll need some traveling companions. Since this is about healing optimally, and you undoubtedly want your journey to be as quick and safe as possible, it only makes sense to have at least one conductor—someone who knows the road well and can guide you at every stage.

The ideal conductor is a medical doctor. Depending on your illness or injury, this may be your primary care doctor or a specialist who is an expert in treating your particular condition. Whomever you choose, it is helpful for you to provide your conductor with your health history. Refer to page 17 for the information that your doctor will need.

Because this is a book on physical healing, and rehabilitation is the cornerstone of this aspect of medicine, you also may want to consult a doctor who is trained in the specialty of physical medicine and rehabilitation (PM&R). As I've mentioned, these doctors—physiatrists—are extremely skilled at helping people travel through the Healing Zone and can work collaboratively with your other doctors to offer you the best plan and resources for recovery.

Physiatrists have special training that involves a 4-year post–medical school program, which they must complete before being able to practice. They also must take both written and oral specialty board examinations.

I remember an incident that occurred while I was on an airplane after taking my oral board exams at the Mayo Clinic in Rochester, Minnesota. The flight attendant announced that a passenger had an urgent need for a doctor. My fellow physiatrists—who also had just completed their exams— and I looked at each other, then one by one pressed our call buttons. As the entire plane lit up, the flight attendant became flustered. A few minutes later she announced, "Is there a doctor on board who is a cardiologist?" What she quickly figured out was that while all doctors are trained to handle medical emergencies, in this instance, the passenger was having a heart attack, and a cardiologist would be the best bet.

While we physiatrists weren't as helpful to the plane passenger as the cardiologist who stepped forward, keep in mind that physiatrists have the most skill and training in helping people with physical recovery. You want the best conductor possible, depending on the situation at hand.

In the rehabilitation model of medicine, physiatrists routinely collaborate with other skilled rehabilitation professionals in a team effort—what we call multidisciplinary care. Working with a team that may include physical and occupational therapists, speech and language pathologists, rehabilitation nurses, and many others helps ensure that you will experience optimal healing. A team approach to rehabilitation is common in most developed countries. The person who should be able to assemble your team is your physiatrist. (See page 20 for a list of rehabilitation professionals.)

Sometimes people try to put their own teams together, with variable results. A woman in the Remarkable Recoveries program at my hospital, Liz Frem, did this following her stroke. Though she received some initial physical therapy and then hired an excellent personal trainer and physical therapist who continued to work with her, she didn't have a conductor in charge of her overall physical recovery.

Liz is intelligent and resourceful, and she progressed nicely despite the absence of a conductor. But about a year after her stroke, she came to see me. I started her on a structured and comprehensive rehabilitation program, which helped her to heal better and more quickly.

As is true for most people who have faced serious illness or injury, the main objective for Liz was to heal *optimally*. When I first saw her, she had done a terrific job of healing to that point. But with a formal rehabilitation program, she was able to make further gains in strength, balance, and coordination, which had an impressive impact on her ability to function day to day. Liz's Remarkable Recovery story appears at the end of this chapter.

INFORMATION THAT YOUR DOCTOR NEEDS

Doctors are taught to write down medical information in a very specific manner. If you fill in this form and hand it to your doctor (or any other health care professional), you will save her a lot of time. Then she can focus on getting you the help that you need now.

History of Present Illness

Your name (including any nickname you like to go by)

_____

Your date of birth

_____

Your age (they can do the math, but it's better if you just write it out)

_____

Whether you are right- or left-handed

_____

The date of onset of your illness or injury

_____

Where you were hospitalized (include the name of each hospital and the dates you were a patient)

_____

_____

_____

The medical problems related to your illness or injury that you are experiencing now

_____

_____

_____

Medications

Your current medications (include over-the-counter drugs and any herbal or nutritional supplements; specify how often you take each one and in what dose)

_____

_____

_____

Allergies

Allergies to medications (write down what happened when you took them in the past)

_____

_____

_____

Past Medical History

Medical conditions, either past or ongoing (not related to your current condition)

_____

_____

_____

Previous surgeries (include the year, if possible)

_____

_____

_____

Family History

Medical conditions that run in your family (include your parents, siblings, and children)

_____

_____

_____

Social History

Describe your home life (e.g., whom you live with; whether your home has stairs)

_____

_____

_____

Describe your work life (e.g., what you do; whether you're retired)

_____

_____

_____

Describe your habits (especially how much alcohol you drink and whether you smoke, now or in the past)

_____

_____

_____

Tests

If you are able to remember the tests you have had, make a note of them. Ideally, you can provide the written reports. Some doctors will want to see the actual films from imaging tests; you might want to inquire about this before your appointment.

_____

_____

_____

Finding the Right Traveling Companions

Prior to having a medical problem, you likely never consulted a physiatrist. If you haven't crossed paths with one by now, you may be wondering how—in the middle of a health crisis—you are supposed to find a doctor who can coordinate all of the various aspects of your healing journey.

Of course, not everyone will have easy access to a doctor who is knowledgeable about physical healing, but the vast majority will if they make a few inquiries. Start with the doctor whom you trust most and ask whether it would be worthwhile for you to see a rehabilitation specialist. Another great resource is a rehabilitation hospital or outpatient center, if there is one near you. The American Academy of Physical Medicine and Rehabilitation, which is the professional organization for physiatrists, also can refer you to a specialist in your area. (See Appendix B on page 239 for contact information.)

While I certainly can't vouch for every doctor in my specialty, I can say that all of us are trained to care for people who are in the Healing Zone. Though our levels of skill and compassion may vary, inviting one of us to travel with you is usually a good idea.

Author Maureen Pratt has been living with systemic lupus erythematosus (lupus for short) for more than a decade. In her spiritually based book, _Peace in the Storm,_ she shares her thoughts on the value of finding the right doctor.

> If you knew of a hidden treasure, you'd probably go to great lengths to find it. Besides following a map (if there was one), you'd keep your ears and eyes open for clues as to its whereabouts and brave any obstacle to get to it. Moreover, you'd follow your

(continued on page 22)

Rehabilitation Professionals

Rehabilitation professionals can be important members of your Super Healing team. They work together in what is known as a multidisciplinary approach to health care. Who will be on your team depends on a number of factors, including what kind of illness or injury you are experiencing. For example, most people in the Healing Zone won't need to consult a speech and language pathologist (SLP). However, an SLP can be incredibly helpful to someone who has suffered a stroke or traumatic brain injury and is experiencing speech or swallowing problems. Your doctor, or conductor, can help you decide which of these professionals should be on your team.

Medical doctor: Usually this is a physiatrist (a doctor specializing in physical medicine and rehabilitation, or PM&R).

Physical therapist: A physical therapist can help someone recover strength, flexibility, endurance, and mobility after illness or injury. This person also treats pain and sometimes manages conditions such as lymphedema. Many physical therapists specialize in certain types of medical conditions (e.g., orthopedic versus neurologic).

Occupational therapist: The primary goal of occupational therapy is to help someone resume routine daily activities, such as bathing and dressing. As a result, occupational therapists devote considerable effort to improving functional use of the arms, including increasing arm strength, coordination, and range of motion. Occupational therapists also are instrumental in assessing skills and prescribing adaptive equipment.

Speech and language pathologist: This type of therapist concentrates on problems that involve language comprehension or expression, as well as issues with swallowing. A speech and language pathologist can offer very simple strategies that will help with speaking and swallowing. Sometimes speech therapists work with people on higher level cognitive activities such as memory, concentration, planning, abstract reasoning, and decision making.

Rehabilitation nurse: These health care specialists perform all of the usual nursing functions but also focus on assisting patients with bowel and bladder function and sexuality issues, as well as providing education and support for the family. Good rehab nurses will help people regain the ability to move, speak, and swallow (among other functions) by reinforcing what the therapy team is working on.

Vocational specialist: This professional evaluates whether someone can return to work and, if so, how best to accomplish it. Sometimes adaptive equipment such as a one-handed computer keyboard is necessary; in other cases, vocational retraining may be recommended so that a person can work in an entirely different occupation.

Therapeutic recreational therapist: The most comprehensive hospitals have at least one therapeutic recreational therapist on staff. This specialist helps people embrace the leisure and educational activities that are part of having a good quality of life, such as cooking, gardening, and playing sports.

Mental health counselor: Most rehabilitation settings will have mental health counseling available. It might involve a consultation with a medical doctor who specializes in psychiatry or perhaps visits with a psychologist or a clinical social worker. These specialists have a lot of experience in helping people make the psychological transition to a life that is likely different than what they previously knew.

Neuropsychologist: This is a specific type of mental health specialist who is responsible for formal testing to determine both obvious and subtle cognitive deficits in people who have had brain injuries (e.g., traumatic brain injuries or strokes).

Registered dietitian: A registered dietitian can be enormously helpful when it comes to figuring out the best diet for someone in the Healing Zone. A dietitian can also offer guidance on how to gain or lose weight, lower cholesterol levels, manage diabetes, and so on.

Orthotist: This person has training in fitting and making braces, which are sometimes necessary for people who have been injured or have paralysis.

Case manager: This person serves as a liaison between the rehabilitation team, the insurance company, the patient, and the patient's family. It can be a tricky job—especially if, for example, an insurance company is not willing to pay for certain treatments. Usually case managers are very helpful in answering your questions and assisting with getting the best possible care. You should always ask who the case manager works for (e.g., the insurance company or the hospital), so you know where his primary allegiance lies. This doesn't mean that he won't be a strong advocate for you, but if issues arise that make you uncomfortable or the case manager does not seem to be a strong advocate for you, then it might be helpful to know who is paying his salary. Most people really appreciate their case managers, who are great at guiding them through a complicated medical process.

intuition, your "sense" of where the treasure might be. You might have to spend a lot of time looking and go out of your way to search. There might be dead ends and disappointments.

But you wouldn't give up until you held the treasure firmly in your hands.

The right doctor is certainly a treasure! Someone who is compassionate and competent, willing to communicate and listen, is to be valued, is worth looking for.

Whether or not you believe that your doctor is a treasure, be sure that he or she is a good conductor, because you'll need one to make this journey as successful as possible. While healing does occur on its own, the right intervention can greatly help facilitate the process and alleviate unnecessary suffering. This certainly is not to suggest that we can eliminate all suffering. But we can address the unnecessary pain, fatigue, and other symptoms that often plague people who are in the process of healing. Finding the right conductor—an expert who has guided many people through physical recovery—can go a long way toward helping you to heal optimally.

One of my patients who is a breast cancer survivor wrote to me when I was ill and offered this insight: "From personal experience, I know the diagnosis is very shocking and frightening. Seek out the best people you can trust in an institution you respect. Together they will get you through this." That's good advice.

Family and Friends

Before we leave the topic of your traveling companions, I want to talk a bit about how loved ones and others who are supportive can help you. Everyone knows that a good support system is extremely useful during any crisis. But did you know that love and support can actually help you heal better and faster? One way to illustrate this point is to take a look at the scientific studies that have been done on mice.

Some strains of mice are monogamous and mate for life, while others are considered polygamous because the male mates with multiple females. In studies involving both strains, monogamous mice that are separated from their partners have delayed rates of wound healing, compared with those that remain with their partners. In the polygamous strains, the social environment does not seem to affect wound healing. Put another way, the freewheeling "bachelor" mice—which don't form strong attachments to any one particular female mouse—don't experience the health benefits of a social environment that promotes wound healing.

Does this mean that humans with loving relationships will heal better? Absolutely, and I'll explore this more extensively in Chapter 11. Because it is so important, I have included "remaining connected to the world and your loved ones" as one of the factors that can positively influence physical healing, as you'll see in the next section. Thus, as you board this train, be sure to take with you those around you who will be loving and supportive.

Understanding Physical Recovery

Now that you know what you need for this healing journey, we're ready to explore how optimal physical healing occurs. Multiple factors play a role in recovery, including the origin and extent of the injury or illness, whether or not it is ongoing, what parts of the body are affected, and what the health of the person was like before becoming ill.

Since there is so much to consider, it makes sense that you can't do just one or two things and then be done. When I was recovering from cancer and its treatment, I had little energy, and I knew that I needed to hone my own healing plan into something manageable. I thought, "What are the most important factors in physical healing, and how can I use them to optimally recover?"

The answer to the first part of this question turned out to be startlingly straightforward. It is the advice handed down from generation to generation: Exercise regularly, eat well, and get enough sleep. Sounds simple, right? Well, not really. Although the concepts are basic, implementing them properly is not so easy—especially when your body isn't feeling all that well. It is important to exercise in a manner that builds your strength and endurance and to eat foods that promote healing. Of course, there are many factors to consider when trying to obtain proper rest during the day (pacing) and at night (sleeping).

In Chapter 1, I described how quickly and easily our bodies can lose strength and become out of shape (deconditioned) as we enter the Healing Zone. But losing strength is only one of the three primary factors within our control that contribute to poor healing. The other two are how you fuel your body and how you allow it to rest. Serious illness almost universally involves not only recovery from the illness itself but also this triad of factors that cause people to heal slowly and poorly. Physical deconditioning, inadequate nutrition, and lousy sleep patterns are what I call the Triple Threat to optimal healing.

The Triple Threat begins at the onset of any serious medical condition. Usually the three factors occur nearly simultaneously and work synergistically to create an environment for, at best, mediocre healing and, at worst, truly unsuccessful physical recovery that leads to unnecessary permanent loss of function and disability. Here's an example of how the Triple Threat plays out.

A patient of mine, whom I'll call Joanne, was diagnosed in her early forties with a medical problem that required a major surgical procedure. She was admitted to the hospital and had nothing to eat prior to her surgery, which took place in the late afternoon. The operation went well, and afterward, she spent a few hours in recovery before being transferred to a room in the regular ward.

Joanne, who had never been hospitalized before, found out what is well documented in the medical literature—that hospitals are noisy and involve frequent interruptions all through the night, leading to extremely poor sleep patterns and a suboptimal healing environment. Joanne didn't like the food and was in considerable pain, so she ate very little. The only time she got up was when she needed to use the bathroom.

Following the current medical model, in which patients are often sent home "quicker and sicker" because of insurance and other health care market influences, Joanne was discharged less than 72 hours after her surgery. By the time she got home, she was well into the Triple Threat. The pattern of not moving around much and not eating or sleeping well was synergistically working against her to greatly impede her physical recovery.

Several weeks after her surgery, the pattern that had begun in the hospital persisted. Joanne felt weak and exhausted, continued to sleep poorly due to both pain and worry, and often was too tired or too disinterested in food to make herself something decent to eat. She returned to work 3 weeks after her operation, but she barely got through the day and collapsed on the couch in the evening. In the morning, she awoke unrefreshed and had trouble starting her day, so she usually skipped breakfast except for her coffee. Her mood plummeted, and she struggled with pain around her incision site. When she went for a follow-up appointment with her surgeon, he didn't seem to find anything unusual about her complaints. He told her to be patient.

The Triple Threat proceeded in this manner: Joanne slept poorly and awakened tired. Because she had no energy, she didn't feel capable of exercise, which led to further loss of strength and endurance. Though she usually ate a fairly nutritious diet, she was skipping meals or grabbing quick snacks. She drank more coffee than usual to give her energy; to help relieve stress and improve her sleep, she got in the habit of drinking one or two glasses of wine in the evenings. The worse Joanne slept, the more her diet deteriorated, and the less willing she was to be physically active. A terrible diet combined with a lack of exercise was the perfect setup for second-rate sleep. Being constantly exhausted prompted Joanne to pay less and less attention to her nutritional needs. Though her body was trying to mend itself, Joanne was trapped in the Triple Threat cycle, which was undermining her ability to heal well.

The good news is that you can take control of the Triple Threat and transform it into three powerful recovery tools, which I call the Super Healing Synergy. This is the exact opposite of the Triple Threat. The combination of the three factors—exercise, diet, and rest—can work powerfully for you or against you. Make them work for you, and you experience the Super Healing Synergy effect in which the three together are far more potent than any one alone.

To illustrate how the Super Healing Synergy works, I'll share with you what one of the doctors in my specialty told me when I was in training: "Knowing how to help someone heal is like knowing how to be a great chef. Let's say you want to make a cake, and you have the core ingredients— flour, sugar, eggs, and oil. You will be able to make a delicious cake only if you have a recipe, you use the right ingredients in the proper amounts, and you bake the cake at the correct temperature for a precise amount of time." What he meant is that even though it seems easy to bake a cake if you have all of the necessary ingredients, it really isn't so simple unless you have more knowledge about how to use them.

Therefore, while on the surface the three factors that have a tremendous effect on physical healing (as well as emotional health) seem relatively basic, in reality they will be extremely useful to you only if you understand just how to incorporate them into your healing plan. I'll discuss each in great detail throughout this book. In the next chapter, I'll outline the Super Healing Plan, which will make it easy for you to implement recovery strategies from each of the three categories.

The Triple Threat also can affect people living with chronic conditions such as arthritis, fibromyalgia, and multiple sclerosis. The combination of poor sleep and suboptimal diet and exercise definitely threatens your ability to physically function as well as possible. But it's difficult to focus on these areas of your life when you're feeling less than your best. If you have a chronic condition, recognizing the Triple Threat can help you to utilize the Super Healing Synergy. This does not mean that you can cure the underlying condition but, rather, that you are optimizing your health status.

Combining All of the Healing Factors

While exercise, diet, and rest are exceedingly important, a number of other factors influence physical healing and also can work synergistically for or against you as you strive to recover. You might think of these as the "spices" that will change your cake from something very plain to an extraordinary confection. They are not the most important to physical healing, but they certainly can affect how well and how quickly you mend. They are:

1. Relieving pain
2. Avoiding prolonged anxiety or depression
3. Considering how spirituality affects health and healing
4. Remaining connected to the world and your loved ones
5. Being able to adjust to having a setback
6. Feeling hopeful about the future

I often think of these, when they are working against someone who's trying to heal, as "collateral damage." When passing through the Healing Zone, it's not at all unusual to feel extremely worried or even depressed. Some people will have unrelenting pain; almost everyone will experience setbacks. It's no surprise, then, that they might withdraw from others and feel less optimistic about the future. This collateral damage impedes healing. But just as you can turn the Triple Threat into a Super Healing Synergy, you can turn this collateral damage into strategies that will enhance your ability to physically recover.

In a fascinating article titled "Connectivity and Healing: Some Hypotheses about the Phenomenon and How to Study It," psychiatrist Lewis Mehl-Madrona, MD, notes that conventional medicine often looks at healing as a linear course when in fact it often is much more complex. An example of a linear course would be a case of pneumonia that is treatable with a short course of antibiotic pills. It's pretty easy to see the cause (bacteria) and the cure (antibiotics) in a linear fashion. But if the patient doesn't respond to the antibiotics and becomes severely ill, she may be hospitalized and require more complicated treatment and a lengthier recovery period. In this scenario, Dr. Mehl-Madrona discusses healing as a process that involves "coherence," which is the coming together of seemingly unrelated behaviors, events, processes, or measurements.

To illustrate coherence, Dr. Mehl-Madrona uses the example of soldiers marching in unison. Imagine their loud and cohesive clomping—a powerful force. It's so powerful, in fact, that it could collapse a bridge. This is why soldiers will break formation and run randomly across a bridge, then resume their formation on the other side. Through this marching metaphor, you can see how the things that I mention in this book can come together and work synergistically to create a far more potent healing force than the more easily understood linear course, which doesn't work well for complicated medical problems.

Your body is quite remarkable in its ability to heal. It will do this regardless of whether or not you help it, but some assistance can improve the ultimate outcome. This means that even if you don't follow the advice in this book, your body will work toward recovery—but providing the best environment possible will help you to heal optimally.

Taking Back Control

Before we move on to the Super Healing Plan, it's important to acknowledge that any change in our health status throws us into a state of turmoil and can make us feel out of control. The purpose of this book is to help you take back some control—step by step. In *Healing Together: How to Bring Peace into Your Life and the World,* author Lee Jampolsky sums it up this way: "To feel powerless is a common human experience because there are some things we obviously have no control over. However, even in situations where we feel such impotence, we can still empower ourselves to take positive action and choose a positive direction." Working toward physical recovery is an important goal that can help take you from powerlessness to empowerment.

While this book is intended to give you the information you need to heal well, please keep in mind that you don't need to do everything perfectly (e.g., eat an ideal diet all the time or adhere to a strict exercise regimen and never miss a workout). In the past, I have described this as the Bill Clinton "one wrong move" rule. Perhaps you recall the March 14, 1997, incident in which then President Clinton arrived at Hobe Sound and was looking forward to a golf excursion later in the day. While heading toward his guest cottage, he descended a flight of stairs, and his heel caught on a step. He stumbled, and as he fell, his leg snapped so loudly that others could hear it. Quite literally, President Clinton took one wrong step.

While one wrong step certainly can cause an injury, there is no such thing in the recovery phase. The rule simply doesn't apply. If you don't exercise regularly, you experience a bout of depression, you like to eat dessert, or you decide that you don't want to tap your spiritual reserves, you still will be able to heal. So don't be concerned if you don't follow all of the guidelines that I set forth in this book. Rather, think of them as a plan to help you take the necessary steps to heal as best you can.

An ancient proverb declares, "If fate throws a knife at you, there are two ways of catching it—by the blade and by the handle." Think of reading this book and following the Super Healing Plan as a way of catching fate's knife by the handle.

REMARKABLE RECOVERY

Liz Frem

In mid-August 2004, Liz Frem—an avid golfer and exercise enthusiast— had just been told by her doctor that she was in the best shape of her life. A few days later, on August 24, she awoke with the worst head- ache of her life. She didn't know it yet, but a blood vessel in her brain was leaking. She was having a stroke.

Liz's previous good health likely contributed to her successful recovery, though it took nearly 2 years. During this time, she experi- enced many of the issues that I discuss in this book, including pain, fatigue, and healing setbacks and plateaus. Nevertheless, Liz perse- vered. Her story is remarkable for the grace and courage she demon- strated throughout. Here is Liz's story, in her words.

Monday night I had a very bad headache, so I went to bed early. I woke up in the middle of the night, felt even worse, even achier. I went to sit up and I fell back. My initial reaction was to laugh, because I just was so silly. I had the headache from hell with blurred vision.

I woke my husband. We called my doctor, who was on vacation. We had no sense of urgency. I thought I might be dizzy from a middle- ear infection. After diddling around for a little while, we decided that we would go to the hospital. In the emergency room the nurse was saying that there is someone in the chair who's had a stroke. I didn't realize that she was talking about me. All of a sudden I became number one on the list. I got whizzed back, and people start coming in. They mentioned the word *stroke* to my husband. I'm still not aware of it. The day is a blur. My family was in shock—this healthy 57-year- old woman had a stroke.

All I wanted to do was get better. I never ever doubted my recovery, and I expected to be better in 6 weeks. I remember the first time my husband took me out for an airing, as we called it, and we went to our place of business. I thought I was doing very well with my walker. I'm sure, in retrospect, that I probably scared most of my employees, because a week or two earlier I was out playing golf and training for a 60-mile walk. Now 60 feet was a major accomplish- ment.

Several months later, I finished physical therapy, but I was having difficulty maneuvering and having dizzy episodes. My headaches were still debilitating, and I wasn't making progress as quickly as I would have liked. I guess for the first time the emotional piece of it hit me, and I hit the wall. I didn't feel that I was far enough along, so I tried other things. My neurologist had suggested yoga, so I went to a couple of yoga classes. It didn't work for me.

A lot of the trouble I was having had to do with stamina. I got very tired. Today my life is better. I'm back. There is very little I cannot do, but I plan my days differently. After rehabilitation, I'd say that I'm about 95 percent of where I was before. Without it, I would probably be at about 70 or 75 percent. Who knows? I may have gotten there because I had found people to help me along the way, but Spaulding certainly made it happen a lot faster and much easier.

There is not a day that goes by that I'm not aware of the fact that I've had a stroke. When I get tired, my right eye droops, and that's never going to go away. I have more difficulty in the evenings, but I'm very good in the morning. Until 3 o'clock you'd never know, and in the evening you might think that I was just tired.

Chapter 3

A Plan to Heal

In *Deep Survival*, journalist Laurence Gonzales tells readers, "The first rule is: Face reality. Good survivors aren't immune to fear. They know what's happening, and it does 'scare the living shit out of' them. It's all a question of what you do next."

Gonzales's book is about surviving natural disasters and other kinds of trauma, not serious illness. However, the principles of survivorship are remarkably similar across the continuum. After surviving a serious illness or injury, the next step is to face reality and decide how you are going to live. Ideally, this will include devising a plan that focuses on physical recovery.

In this chapter, I'll give you the framework for a healing plan. You can tailor it, with the help of your health care team, to fit your personal situation and needs. As I describe this plan, keep in mind that it will work best for you if you evaluate your current health status, create realistic goals, and review them with your doctor.

Mapping a Route from Fear to Hope

There is something very reassuring about having a plan. A plan will help you not only to physically heal better but also to weather the emotional part of your journey. Fear is a common denominator in nearly every cancer survivor's travels through the Healing Zone. This is true of people with many other diagnoses as well.

Remember crime victim Sasha Kondratiuk, whom I mentioned in the introduction? It's easy to see why fear would be a significant factor in her recovery. At the end of this chapter is her Remarkable Recovery story. This is what Sasha has to say about how she dealt with her fear.

> From a psychological point of view, it was important for me to accept the fact that going outside in public again would take

time, and I could not go back to walking around by myself in a city for a while. For months, all I could handle doing was walking across the street from my mother's apartment to the bakery/ coffee shop. Although this does not seem like a big deal, physically and psychologically for me to do that on my own was huge. I think these types of "small wins" were really important for me to realize that I was in fact making progress and healing.

It's difficult not to be afraid when you face a health crisis, but it's important to try to avoid letting fear get in the way of your ability to heal. As Frances Moore Lappé and Jeffrey Perkins, authors of *You Have the Power,* suggest, "Maybe we can never hope to leave fear behind, but by being willing to take the first leap, we put ourselves in motion. Our fears become linked to goals that really matter to us, and we take heart in witnessing our own movement."

Creating a healing plan is forward movement in your journey. It is also part of transitioning from critical illness to better health. Yet there is no doubt that transitions are filled with uncertainty and make us feel uncomfortable.

In his book *The Way of Transition,* William Bridges discusses how transitions, which are an inevitable part of a serious illness experience, alter one's previous reality—so much so that even though the medical condition is only one facet of our lives, it seems to change everything. Bridges, who has spent many years studying how transitions affect people, writes that "if it is deep and far-reaching, transition makes a person feel that not only is a piece of reality gone, but that everything that has seemed to be reality was simply an enchantment. With the spell broken, life can look so different that we hardly recognize it."

Bridges makes an interesting distinction between "transition" and "change," proffering that most people resist the former rather than the latter. Indeed, it is transition that makes us feel worried and wary. Unfortunately, there is no getting around it—your time spent in the Healing Zone is a period of transition. During this time, some people become immobilized by fear and uncertainty. Others will take that negative energy and use it to help them recover. Bridges sums it up this way: "Transition helps you come to terms with change. It reorients you so that you can mobilize your energy to deal successfully with your new situation . . . instead of being hampered by attitudes and behaviors that were developed for and more appropriate to your old situation."

Creating a healing plan encourages you to view your current situation in a new light in order to determine how best to resolve or come to terms with physical limitations. It helps create order out of disordered and changed circumstances. Or, as Wendy Schlessel Harpham, MD (who has spent years in and out of treatment for lymphoma), writes, "Out of yesterday's rubble, I had to find or create a new normal for today and a renewed faith in tomorrow."

Cindi Broaddus knows a lot about transitions and the need to create a new normal out of yesterday's rubble. You may recall hearing about a particularly horrific crime in which Cindi (who is related to talk-show host Dr. Phil McGraw) was terribly burned by acid that someone had thrown off a highway overpass at the car she was riding in below. In her book *A Random Act,* she describes her healing journey, which involved many personal choices. Cindi writes, "First, I decided what kind of survivor I would choose to be. Second, I made the choice to heal from the inside out. And finally, I chose what to do with the rest of my life."

For everyone who faces a serious medical condition, the road to healing is filled with choices, and making a commitment to spend the time on recovery is important. As you travel through the Healing Zone, you'll find that all along the way there will be crossroads—different paths you can take. It isn't necessarily that one path is right and all the rest are wrong; rather, there are simply multiple ways that you can approach your recovery based on a variety of factors, including your condition and your personality and philosophy.

Keep in mind that while I will encourage you to develop a plan and to set goals, the Bill Clinton "one wrong move" rule does not apply—which means, thankfully, that you don't need to be perfect to heal well.

Setting Goals

In the rehabilitation model of medicine, setting goals is paramount. If you don't define what you want to achieve, then it's difficult to accomplish any given task. Goals offer you a way to measure where you are now and visualize what you want to achieve in the future. Or, as the infamous baseball icon Yogi Berra once said, "If you don't know where you are going, you might wind up someplace else."

Setting the right goals is essential for success. Goals give structure and purpose to your healing plan. A healing journey without goals is akin to driving on an unpaved path, whereas goals steer you onto a paved road.

You can Super Heal without goals, but it's far easier to accomplish something if you know what it is that you want. As Fyodor Dostoevsky wrote in *The Brothers Karamazov,* "The secret of man's being is not only to live, but to have something to live for." We could translate this into a modern-day healing mantra and say, "The secret of healing is not just hoping for recovery but working with a purpose."

Though it's impossible to tell what someone might be able to achieve in 1 month, much less 1 year, setting goals is an important first step. Because recovery is not entirely predictable, goals should be flexible and the ability to meet them altered as necessary. At the medical center where I work, we set short-term and long-term goals for people who are undergoing therapy. I have created the Super Healing Plan to follow this model.

In this plan, you set monthly short-term goals in several categories, as well as biannual (6-month) long-term goals in each of the categories. The Super Healing Plan lasts for 1 year, though you can repeat it at the end of 12 months if you still have the potential for further recovery. So for each category over the course of the year, you will set 12 short-term goals and 2 long-term goals.

While this might seem like a lot of goals, it's actually very easy to do. The only goals you need to worry about initially are the first ones you write down and tackle. Then, at specific intervals, you create new goals (every month for short-term goals and at the 6-month mark for long-term goals). It's a good idea to post your goals on the refrigerator or write them on an index card to carry with you.

I know that not everyone who reads this book will be able to follow the entire plan. I encourage you to read every chapter and glean the information from it that can help you to recover. On page 237, I present the Super Healing Shortcut Plan, which is a good way to get started if you can't do everything. However, I would encourage you to attempt to complete the whole plan and really become engaged in your healing journey.

Here is a summary of the Super Healing Plan.

Main Points

☐ The plan lasts for 12 months and can be repeated.

☐ Short-term goals are set once a month in eight categories (eight short-term goals to start, then eight new goals each month).

☐ Long-term goals are set twice during the plan—once at the beginning and again at the halfway mark, after 6 months (so eight long-term goals to start, then eight new goals at the beginning of the 7th month).

Goal Categories

☐ Exercising in a Therapeutic Manner

☐ Eating a Healing Diet

☐ Obtaining Proper Rest and Sleep

☐ Alleviating Pain

☐ Avoiding Mood Problems

☐ Using Your Mind to Heal Your Body

☐ Improving Loving Relationships and Social Connections

☐ Harnessing Your Spiritual Energy

Plan Your Work and Work Your Plan

As you read this book, I'll offer suggestions about goals that I hope you will find helpful. The tables beginning on page 38 are templates for how you can write down and structure your goals. The examples are just suggestions; they are not necessarily the goals that you should aim to achieve.

As I mentioned before, what I have found in my clinical practice is that people are extremely intelligent about their bodies. They tend to have a good sense of what they can accomplish and what they can't. In creating goals for yourself, I encourage you to consider my suggestions but also talk with your health care team and trust your own instincts—what I sometimes call the "voice of your body."

Reading this book is the beginning of your Super Healing journey. Congratulate yourself on getting off to a good start. Next, set a start date for yourself. Ideally, your start date should be after you've read this book, so you can set appropriate goals. For example, if you think it will take you a week to read this book, then launch your Super Healing Plan next week.

As you read each chapter, keep up the momentum by writing down an initial short-term and long-term goal. There is no better time to begin than today. As it says in the Bible, "If you wait until the wind and the weather are just right, you will never plant anything and never harvest anything" (Eccles. 11:4). A more modern version of this idea came from General George S. Patton, who said, "A good plan violently executed right now is far better than a perfect plan executed next week."

In the Broadway musical *The IT Girl,* the lead actress sings about having the perfect plan to land the man of her dreams. Perfect plans exist only in our imaginations. In real life, there is no perfect plan, which is why you'll need to check your goals every month and adjust them according to your progress. If you don't meet one or more of your goals, it isn't a failure; it's a normal part of the process. Take the time to analyze why you didn't meet a particular goal and make appropriate adjustments to your Super Healing Plan.

As you devise and revise your goals, consider what you want to accomplish and how best to go about it. In short, work on having a vision for your Super Healing Plan. Your vision will evolve as you read the rest of this book and talk with your doctors. However, it helps to be able to see where you want to go in order to get there.

Florence Chadwick learned this when she decided that she would become the first woman ever to swim across the English Channel. For years she trained, and in 1952, she was ready to try. She began full of hope, surrounded by people in small boats who encouraged her to keep going. As she neared the coast of England, she encountered a heavy fog and increasingly cold and choppy waters. Finally, just a few hundred yards from her goal, she gave up and asked to be pulled into a boat. Florence was heartbroken and later said to reporters, "I'm not offering excuses, but I think I could have made it if I had been able to see my goal."

Though defeated once, Florence decided to try again. The second time around, she concentrated on developing a mental image of the coast of England—her finish line. She had a goal and a clear vision for where she wanted to be at the end of her journey. This time, she made it.

Making Healing a Priority

I'm often asked a very basic but extremely important question, which goes something like this: "Dr. Silver, how do you get people to begin to heal when they are so sick and everything is a huge effort?" My answer is that I don't "get" people to do anything. I may inform them and encourage them, but ultimately, each person has to take responsibility for his or her own healing journey. What I have found, however, is that once someone begins, the process becomes much easier and flows nicely.

You may be thinking that you simply can't add one more thing to your list of responsibilities. The prospect of setting goals may seem very overwhelming. Before adding new goals—and thus new responsibilities—to your daily routine discourages you, consider two points.

First, the process of setting goals allows you to accomplish what matters most to you. This is because defining goals assists you in deciding what is most important for you to concentrate on. What is most deserving of your time and attention as you move through this healing experience?

Second, you may find that setting goals actually gives you more time rather than less. By choosing what to focus on, you also are making a decision about what is *not* a priority in your life right now. As I often tell my patients, what I really am saying is that they have "permission" to avoid doing all the boring and physically tiring things they did before they were sick, so they can concentrate on what means the most to them—physically and emotionally.

In the next chapter, I talk more about what it means to take the time to heal, because taking that time is an amazing gift that you give yourself and your loved ones. Even if you feel a bit discouraged right now or find the idea of setting goals somewhat daunting, just by continuing to read, you are moving in the right direction on your healing journey. As the great physician and poet Dr. Oliver Wendell Holmes once said, "The greatest thing in the world is not so much where we are, but in which direction we are moving."

REMARKABLE RECOVERY

Sasha Kondratiuk

On July 5, 2005, I was randomly attacked on the street as I was walking home from work. It was around 8:00 p.m. and still light out, since it was summer. A man began following me a couple of blocks away from my apartment in Washington, DC. I tried to sprint away as fast as I could, but he ran after me. When I realized he was in fact running after me—and worse, I saw the man had a knife—I tried to get into the passenger seat of a moving car, but it was locked or I was too panicked to get in. I then suffered a massive blow to my head and collapsed. I was beaten badly and stabbed 11 times—on my back, arm, face, ear, and stomach.

I screamed out for help, yelling that I would be killed if no one helped. I was so lucky to ultimately be saved by people that did help. Otherwise, I certainly would have been killed. My attacker was on PCP, so he was virtually indestructible. When someone hit him with a metal pole, he didn't even flinch. Even when people were fighting him to get him away from me, for some reason he did not fight them, but was intent to get back to me to hurt or kill me for no reason. He never wanted my money or anything, just to hurt me.

I was rushed to George Washington University Hospital in an ambulance. There was blood absolutely everywhere, but the scary thing was that I could not move or feel anything below my waist. When I got to the hospital, I remember asking one of the doctors whether I would live, and the doctor saying he didn't know but he hoped so. One of the deep stab wounds on my back caused a spinal cord injury. Luckily, beyond that in terms of my vital organs, only my liver was damaged, but that was repaired and was able to regenerate and fix itself. Almost all the tendons in my right arm were severed, so I could not move it for weeks. In fact, I couldn't really move anything for weeks while I was in the hospital.

When I was in the rehab hospital, first in Washington, DC, and then in Boston, where my family lives, I did both occupational and physical therapy for a few hours each day. I did physical rehab to attempt to strengthen the left side of my body below the waist, which I was virtually unable to move. I did a lot of exercises, and also electrical stimulation to the muscles I could not move to try to tense them through the electric shocks. For occupational therapy, I learned to use assistive devices to help me bathe and dress myself. I continue physical therapy and the electrical stimulation today to help strengthen my hips and legs. Psychologically, I spoke to a therapist about once a week and then once every 2 weeks to generally discuss my state of mind and how I was dealing with post-traumatic stress disorder.

I healed slowly and incrementally. I went from a state of not being able to move any part of my body to being told I would never walk again and I'd be in a wheelchair for the rest of my life. However, after 3 months, I progressed to using a walker for short distances. Now I walk with only one crutch for long distances.

What helped me is my mind and the amazing ability of the human body to rehabilitate itself. For a long time, and to an extent even today, the whole experience felt so surreal—like it could not possibly have happened to me. I think this sort of detachment helped me move forward full force to do everything I could in my physical rehab. I really pushed myself because mentally I knew that I had to, and I was able to dissociate from the monumental task of facing my rehab.

Remaining positive about any progress, no matter how small, was also important to keep me motivated to work hard. I think being realistic about progress is so important, because it is really easy to compare "before" and "after" and get upset about the things you can't do anymore. Although it can be hard to be excited about very little improvements, I think it is so important to celebrate and be driven by those, because they provide hope for bigger improvements.

The most important thing I learned is that individuals must take charge of their recovery. What that meant for me was taking the lead in researching my condition, asking a lot of questions of all my doctors and therapists, looking into alternative therapies, and discussing other individuals' experience with them. It really just means managing every aspect, because no one will be able to manage things as well as you will.

SHORT-TERM GOALS

Begin your Super Healing Plan by choosing a start date. Then, as you read this book, create eight short-term goals—one for each category below. These goals should be ones that you think you can achieve over the next month. The goals I have listed here are just examples and are not intended

	EATING A HEALING DIET	EXERCISING IN A THERAPEUTIC MANNER	OBTAINING PROPER REST AND SLEEP	ALLEVIATING PAIN	
Month 1	Eat 3 meals a day without skipping breakfast.	Obtain a pedometer and track how many steps I take in a day. Then increase this number by 1,000 steps per day by the end of the month.	Give up taking naps, but rest every afternoon by reading a book or listening to music for 30 minutes.	Make an appointment to talk to my doctor about my pain.	
Month 2					
Month 3					
Month 4					
Month 5					
Month 6					
Month 7					
Month 8					
Month 9					
Month 10					
Month 11					
Month 12					

to be a starting point for you. If there is a goal category that you don't feel comfortable with right now or you can't do for some reason, then just skip it. This is your Super Healing Plan, so aim to create goals that you think you can accomplish and that you feel good about. At the end of the month, check your progress and write new short-term goals for the next month.

	AVOIDING MOOD PROBLEMS	USING YOUR MIND TO HEAL YOUR BODY	IMPROVING LOVING RELATIONSHIPS AND SOCIAL CONNECTIONS	HARNESSING YOUR SPIRITUAL ENERGY
	Stop drinking alcohol, which is a depressant.	Meditate every morning for 10 minutes.	Meet a friend once a week for lunch.	Pray most nights before bed.

LONG-TERM GOALS

At the start of your Super Healing Plan, you'll create eight long-term goals. They should be goals that you think you can accomplish over a period of 6 months. Every month when you write new short-term goals, you can review your long-term goals, too. If for any reason they don't seem realistic, come up with new ones. It's fine to change your goals; the point is to have them

	EATING A HEALING DIET	EXERCISING IN A THERAPEUTIC MANNER	OBTAINING PROPER REST AND SLEEP	ALLEVIATING PAIN	
Month 1	Eat 5 fruit/vegetable servings each day.	Walk at least 5,000 steps every day.	Sleep at least 7 hours each night.	Follow my doctor's recommendation and go to PT to help with my back pain.	
Month 7					

and focus on healing optimally. At the 6-month mark, you'll set new long-term goals. At the end of a year, if you think you still have room to improve your health, start the Super Healing Plan all over again and write new short-term and long-term goals.

	AVOIDING MOOD PROBLEMS	USING YOUR MIND TO HEAL YOUR BODY	IMPROVING LOVING RELATIONSHIPS AND SOCIAL CONNECTIONS	HARNESSING YOUR SPIRITUAL ENERGY
	Meet with my psychologist regularly once a week.	Meditate for 15 minutes twice a day.	Join a community group and participate in the group's activities.	Take time to pray at least once a day.

Chapter 4

A Time to Heal

In this chapter, I want to focus on something that you can control on your healing journey: time. Without proper time management, your train can derail.

Healing takes time—usually a lot of it. Recovering optimally with a focused plan takes more time than mending without a plan. However, taking time to heal can be a tremendous challenge as you struggle to balance real life with Healing Zone priorities. Many people who are in the process of recovering feel as though they are in limbo—not able to live as they did before while simultaneously not able to devote all of their time and energy to healing.

Katherine Russell Rich is a soft-spoken woman who is instantly likable. After being diagnosed with breast cancer, she took a rough but successful journey through the Healing Zone and eventually wrote about what it was like to live in what she described as two different time zones. One time zone was focused on medical treatment and recovery, while the other—essentially, her former life—continued as though everything was the same as it always had been. Describing this phenomenon in her book *The Red Devil*, Rich wrote:

> In Cancerland . . . people are forced to live in two time zones at once. We exist on cancer's time and real-world time simultaneously. We continue to care about our love lives and careers and vacations and retirement plans—about the big and the small—but with particular urgency, since the clock is racing, double time.

I remember many occasions when I was in the Healing Zone and real life got in the way of my recovery and vice versa. I wanted to focus exclusively on healing, while at the same time I wanted to devote myself to my loved ones.

In my book *After Cancer Treatment: Heal Faster, Better, Stronger,* I share a story about my daughter, who has a life-threatening egg allergy. Shortly after I started chemotherapy, her preschool teacher thought it would be safe to allow her to stir, but not eat, a mixture containing egg. I received an urgent call from her teacher telling me that my daughter was in the middle of a severe allergic reaction. Despite the fact that I felt physically terrible myself, I jumped in the car (with my husband driving) to pick up my daughter and get her to the doctor as quickly as possible.

When she was in kindergarten and I was feeling much better, she had another reaction. This time, the school nurse called to say that 10 chicks had hatched in my daughter's classroom and just breathing the air had set off a severe allergic reaction. Once again, I rushed to the school to get her. Though the situation was similar to the one a couple of years before, there is no doubt that it was a lot easier to manage when I was healthier.

I should mention that my daughter has been blessed with terrific teachers, and the two women in this story are truly wonderful. It can be very difficult to know ahead of time what someone with a severe allergy will react to. This is especially true for a very young child, as it isn't always clear what she can and can't be exposed to.

Of course, during the first allergic episode, it would have been great if I could have said, "I'm having my own crisis right now; let's schedule my daughter's for a more convenient time." (Or better yet, let's not allow her to have any crises at all.) But life doesn't work that way. Things happen to us and to our loved ones that need immediate attention. Sometimes we find ourselves in the midst of more than one drama at a time. It would be great to compartmentalize life's traumas so that they occur sequentially rather than concurrently, but it doesn't always work that way. So taking the time to heal doesn't mean that the real world disappears. Most of the time you will be operating in two time zones.

It isn't only crises that make us pay attention to real-world issues. As I was healing, the day-to-day challenges were always present. I was constantly thinking about whether I should focus on what I needed to do or what my children needed me to do. When I returned to work, I faced even more challenges as I tried to finish healing while at the same time doing my job. There isn't an easy solution for living in these two time zones, so I did what I had to do: I compromised. I tried to stay focused on my efforts to heal, but sometimes they fell by the wayside as I lived my real life with real people who had immediate and pressing needs.

One of my patients, Jeff Card, whose Remarkable Recovery story appears at the end of this chapter, struggled throughout his healing journey to live and work in both time zones. He is a brilliant accountant who works for a prestigious firm in Boston. As a vice president, he oversees a huge staff and travels incessantly. While to the outside world he appeared to be doing a fabulous job of balancing working and healing, he is the first to admit that it wasn't easy. It rarely is. But it's necessary.

When Time Is Worth More Than Money

Of the thousands of seriously ill people I have treated, the one thing nearly all of them want is more time. Sometimes this needs a little translation. When people say they want more time, it may be that what they really may want is more energy to accomplish the things they desire. Time and energy are interrelated, and a gain in one often leads to a gain in the other. In fact, time and energy are two of the most important commodities for everyone.

In 1908, Arnold Bennett wrote *How to Live on 24 hours a Day,* which became a bestseller in the United States and England. In this book, Bennett described time as "the ideal democracy." He wrote:

> In the realm of time there is no aristocracy of wealth, and no aristocracy of intellect. Genius is never rewarded by even an extra hour a day. . . . The chief beauty about the constant supply of time is that you cannot waste it in advance. . . . The next year, the next day, the next hour are lying ready for you, as perfect, as unspoilt, as if you had never wasted a single moment in all your career.

I think of taking time to heal as a literal investment in your health. After all, for many people, time is money; spending your hours on physical recovery means you have less in the bank. But it's a great investment. Think about how much you'd be willing to pay if you could upgrade your health. Chances are it's quite a lot. Many people might say that health is priceless.

Of course, you can't simply write a check to improve your health. But you can invest your time and any other necessary resources in achieving this goal. Just as you would with any major life decision, it's important to think through and then make a commitment to taking the time you will need to mend.

As you ponder this decision, consider what Wayne Muller wrote about time and money in his book *Sabbath: Finding Rest, Renewal, and Delight in Our Busy Lives.*

> The point is not that money is bad. Money allows us to participate in the national marketplace and to purchase all the basic goods and services we cannot provide for ourselves. But

how much time should we trade for it? How do we decide when we have too much time and not enough money, and when do we know we have too much money and not enough time? In our culture we so overvalue money that this question is rarely asked. . . . People who have a lot of money and no time, we call 'rich.' And people who have a great deal of time but no money, we call 'poor.' . . . What if we were to expand our definition of wealth to include those things that grow only in time—time to walk in the park, time to take a nap, time to play with children, to read a good book, to dance, to put our hands in the garden, to cook playful meals with friends, to paint, to sing, to meditate, to keep a journal. What if we were to live, for even a few hours, without spending money, cultivating time instead as our most precious resource?

Let's look at how Muller's words can help shape your Super Healing Plan.

Taking Time to Nurture Yourself

It isn't easy to give yourself permission to take the time to heal. You probably have a lot of responsibilities and people counting on you. The fact is, most of us are better at nurturing others than at nurturing ourselves.

For example, during the time that I was writing this chapter, I gave a speech at a cancer fund-raiser. This event was at a hotel and included a spa day for attendees. When I talked with the women who came, all of them felt good about spending the money on pampering; it was, after all, going to a worthy cause. These same women, though, told me that they wouldn't normally take the time or spend the money to nurture themselves with facials, manicures, and massages. This spa day was on the "approved" list because its true purpose was to nurture others—people with cancer—rather than themselves.

Men and women—but particularly women, according to the research—have not learned the skill of self-nurture. Sigmund Freud considered self-nurture a form of narcissism that was infantile and pathologic. But times have changed; we now understand that people who love themselves are much better at loving others than those who don't. Another way of saying this is that you will be better at nurturing those who need you if you nurture yourself first.

In her book *Crossroads at Midlife*, psychologist Frances Cohen Praver, PhD, presents a more modern view of narcissism and nurture. She writes:

A shift in attitudes finds that contemporary analytic thinkers value narcissism as a healthy aspect of mature behavior. We now refer to narcissism as high self-esteem, which inspires expression of the self. . . . Healthy narcissism facilitates aspirations and goals.

Though a shift has taken place in the field of psychology regarding the concept of self-nurture, it hasn't necessarily translated into individuals becoming better at taking care of themselves. Alice Domar, PhD, is an assistant professor of medicine at Harvard Medical School. In her ground-breaking book *Self-Nurture: Learning to Care for Yourself as Effectively as You Care for Everyone Else,* she writes:

> The capacity to self-nurture starts with our relationship with our parents. . . . As children, did we learn the value of self-love and self-care? Did our mothers and fathers present themselves as strong role models of self-nurturance, or were they ceaseless models of self-sacrifice, self-doubt, self-neglect, or even self-abuse?

One of my patients, a woman I'll call Joan, is a classic example of someone who is terrific at nurturing others and not very good at taking care of herself. Joan was diagnosed with breast cancer and needed surgery, followed by chemotherapy. After she finished chemo, while she was still bald and feeling quite ill, she decided to return to work full-time. She came to see me a few days later in tears. She said, "I thought I could handle this, but I can't. I'm too sick, and I start radiation treatment next week!"

I was curious about what prompted Joan to go back to work in such a frail state, with another round of toxic therapy coming up. I assumed that she was worried about losing her job or her family needing her salary. Neither was the case. In fact, she told me that she was receiving her full salary, and no one had put any pressure on her to return. Instead, as someone who constantly nurtured others, she was having a hard time not being able to do this. At the office, she noted, "people count on me." So she decided to go back, even though physically she didn't feel ready.

As I talked with Joan, she realized that her colleagues were getting along just fine without her. They missed her, of course, and when she was there, they had less work to do. But they were willing to support her. Joan recognized that she needed to take the time to finish her treatment and heal so that she could return to her job and be productive and helpful. She needed to nurture herself—or, as some psychologists say, to engage in a "healthy selfishness."

Psychology professors Richard Heller, PhD, and Rachael Heller, PhD, define healthy selfishness as "a way of thinking and acting in which there is a deep appreciation, compassion, and concern for yourself—by yourself. It includes (but is not limited to) your willingness to: respect your feelings, sensitivities, preferences, desires, and needs; trust your knowledge, ability, and experience; accept your weaknesses and imperfections without blame or guilt; encourage your effort and struggles, without demand for success; and offer unconditional love and nurturing of the child within."

Pamper, Please

While you are in the Healing Zone, you'll have to focus on yourself in a loving and nurturing manner. At times, this will mean putting yourself first; what you need must take precedence over what others need. This isn't easy to do if you've been taught, as many of us have, that we should be more concerned with others than with ourselves.

Sometimes it's easier to embrace self-nurturing if you consider the opposite option: self-denial. Drs. Heller and Heller define self-denial as "the surrendering of your needs, preferences, and desires in order to fulfill the needs, preferences, or desires of another person." Though chronic self-denial is unhealthy, it is particularly problematic if you are recovering from a serious illness or injury. This is truly a time when your focus should first and foremost be on helping yourself to heal.

If you find it difficult to take the time to nurture yourself, you are in good company. Many wonderful people are not good self-nurturers. Nevertheless, it's important to try to change this as you mend. Begin with small steps. Reading this book is a terrific start. Next, find the time to make a plan to heal, as I outlined in the previous chapter. There is no doubt that illness provides opportunities, and one of them is a chance to reflect on how to take better care of ourselves.

If you haven't spent much time nurturing yourself in the past, psychiatrist Edward Hallowell, MD, believes that you can change. He suggests, "If you never taught yourself how to tend to yourself—if, indeed, you were taught to ignore your needs and feelings as if they were selfish and impure—it is still possible to learn how to make a healthy connection to yourself."

It's easy to avoid self-nurture. As relationship expert Susan Page explains:

> The insidious thing about not taking care of yourself is that if you don't do it, no one else in the world may ever notice. If you don't feed your children and buy them clothes and support them when they need your help, they'll notice. If you don't keep your agreements with your partner, your partner will be unhappy and will let you know. But you can fail to take care of yourself and your own needs for years, and no one will care. . . .

Of course, great excuses are plentiful: I don't have time. I keep forgetting. I'll do it later. I *am* going to do it—but not yet. The best excuse of all is, taking care of myself is not as important as all the other things I have to do—for other people.

During your time in the Healing Zone, self-nurture is something to strive for. Here are examples of ways in which you can nurture yourself.

- Listen to music, talk radio, audiobooks, or a relaxation tape.
- Meditate or pray.
- Watch television.
- Read a book or magazine.
- Sit down and talk with someone in person or on the phone.
- Perform deep breathing and relaxation exercises.
- Play a game on the computer or with a friend.
- Play a musical instrument.
- Crochet, macramé, knit, needlepoint, or sew.
- Make a craft or jewelry.
- Carve wood.
- Scrapbook.
- Do a jigsaw or crossword puzzle.
- Draw or paint a picture.
- Write a letter, e-mail, journal entry, or poem or short story.
- Sit in a comfortable place with a warm drink (decaffeinated and non-alcoholic is best).
- Lie down and take time to reflect.
- Go for a scenic drive.
- Sit outside or take a walk someplace where you can enjoy nature.
- Go for a manicure, pedicure, massage, or another spa treatment.
- Exercise.

I can't tell you how to balance your responsibilities in the time zones of real life and recovery, but I can encourage you to simply do the best that you can. Try to stay focused on healing, but also recognize that it's okay to take some breaks and do what you need to do in the real world. Keep in mind that the better you heal and the more strength and energy you have, the easier it will be for you to resume your former responsibilities and care for those who depend on you. As William Shakespeare observed, "Self-love, my liege, is not so vile a sin as self-neglecting."

Prioritizing and Pacing

There is a story about a man who seeks enlightenment. He travels a great distance to consult a Zen master. The master invites the man to tea and fills his cup to the brim. Every time the man takes a drink, the master refills the cup to the point where it overflows onto the saucer. The master is silent all the while, until finally the man—who is becoming increasingly exasperated—asks the master why he doesn't say anything but just keeps pouring tea. The master responds, "Your cup is too full. You keep adding to it, and now it is overflowing. There is no room for enlightenment until you empty your cup."

This is true of healing optimally as well. If your life is bursting at the seams, you won't have the time or the energy to recover as well as possible. You'll need to empty your cup a bit to make room to heal.

Making time to focus on healing can certainly be challenging, but one thing that really helps is to prioritize your daily activities. In the previous chapter, we reviewed goals—why they are important and how to set them. But goals become meaningless if you don't take the time to achieve them. Goals are a powerful (and usually an essential) way to successfully travel through the Healing Zone. As you consider and plan your goals, keep in mind that you want to be devoting the maximum amount of time in your day to those things that will help you to heal. If you don't do this, and instead spend your time running your body into the ground by working too much or too hard or doing too many errands or chores, you likely won't be able to heal optimally.

Just as time and energy are inextricably linked, so are prioritizing and pacing. The late Hugh Gallagher, a polio survivor and Franklin Roosevelt biographer, once wrote, "My muscle power and endurance are as coins in my purse: I have only so many and they will buy only so much. I must live within my means, and to do this I have to economize: what do I want to buy and how can I buy it for the least possible cost?"

Everyone has limited "coins." In the Healing Zone, many people have fewer than they did in the past. In order to reach your goals, you will need to use your muscle power and endurance wisely.

Healing well is not about pushing yourself to the limit without consideration for what tasks are important or how they will affect your body. It requires a more thoughtful approach in which you set goals and modify your activities to achieve those goals. While healing well does include physically challenging your body to improve strength and endurance, it also involves periods of relaxation and rest. In short, in order to heal well, you need to prioritize and pace.

Everyone should prioritize and pace, but when you are in the Healing Zone, this becomes particularly important. When I talk with my patients about these concepts, they often jump to the conclusion that I am telling them not to do the things that they enjoy. In fact, that's not what I'm recommending. Instead, think of it as your chance to unload all of the boring and tedious tasks that you never enjoyed doing anyway. This has been a societal trend for a number of years. We now have ways to order tickets to events without standing in line, to buy groceries without ever going to the supermarket, to get our clothes dry-cleaned by setting a bag filled with dirty garments outside the front door, and so on. You have many options for trimming your to-do list while at the same time maintaining the time and energy to do what brings you pleasure.

Regardless of whether you decide to hire people and enlist various services, this is a good time to let friends know how they can help. You certainly can do this in a very considerate way that will not overly burden those close to you. For example, find out when your friend is next going grocery shopping, and ask whether he could pick up a few items for you at the same time. Or ask a co-worker to pick up lunch for you when she goes out for a break.

If you consider your daily activities prior to your illness or injury, you'll likely find plenty of things you did in the past that simply don't need to be done at all, or at least not in the same way. For example, while I would not advise anyone to skip bathing altogether, switching from a daily shower to an every-other-day routine is a great way to conserve energy.

Pacing Basics

There are a few basic principles when it comes to pacing. These may seem obvious, but as you read them, ask yourself whether you are doing them. If not, they are good tools to use in the recovery process.

1. Organize and plan your day ahead of time. This is very important, though it will cost you up front. This goes back to priorities. Skip the things that aren't that meaningful or cause you to be overly fatigued. Include those things that support your recovery or bring you pleasure. If you need to do something that you know will be tiring (e.g., painting your home or doing your taxes), spread it out over several days or even weeks. Better yet, ask someone else to do it for you.

Try to exercise early in the day, when your energy level is highest. Of course, this may not work for everyone's schedule. Exercise is important enough that you should make time for it even if it needs to be later in the day. Keep in mind that exercising right before bedtime can contribute to poor sleep.

2. Plan and take breaks (rest periods). This doesn't mean you have to take a nap. I recommend napping only if you are sleeping well at night and still feel exhausted during the day. If you aren't sleeping well at night and you nap during the day, it sets up a vicious cycle of poor sleep. Most people don't need to nap and would do better with an earlier bedtime or a later wake-up time—or both.

However, planning breaks during the day is important to give your body and your mind a rest. You should find time to sit down in a comfortable chair and read, listen to music, meditate, or do whatever you find relaxing. Depending on your energy level, stage of recovery, current treatment regimen, and work and family commitments, you may need to be creative about when and how you take breaks. But do it. Put up your feet and be good to yourself.

3. Use good body mechanics. Poor body mechanics are a huge energy drain. Sitting at your computer in a chair that is not supportive and doesn't have armrests (sometimes called data arms, if they attach to the desk and are not part of the chair) is very taxing. Standing (and bending over) while doing household chores such as cooking, folding laundry, washing the car, and gardening also is very tiring. Don't mistake activities such as these for exercise. These tasks will do little to build your strength and endurance, so you should conserve your energy while performing them.

4. Set your thermostat at a comfortable temperature. Some of my friends take great pride in waiting until a certain predetermined date to turn on their heat or air-conditioning, despite the outdoor temperature. It's great to be frugal and to be conscious of the environment. However, it takes a lot of extra energy for you to keep your body warm or cool. Living or working in an environment that's too cold or too hot will unnecessarily sap your energy. It also is wise to avoid exercising in extreme heat or cold.

5. Avoid straining or pushing yourself to the point of exhaustion. I tell my patients to listen to the "voice" of their bodies. What is your body telling you? Are your legs or arms getting tired? Are you feeling more pain? Are you having trouble concentrating? All of these are warning signs that you are pushing too hard. Try to heed these signals right away so you don't reach the point of severe exhaustion or pain.

Your Energy Inventory

Before you begin to really pace yourself, it is a good idea to spend 3 days keeping track of what you are doing. After all, one of the best ways to see how you can save your time and energy "coins" is to first see how you are spending them.

I advise my patients to keep a 3-day log of their activities. They write down everything that they do, along with when they are experiencing pain or feeling particularly fatigued. Here's what to do.

1. Organize a notebook with space to write in for each hour of the day for 3 days.

2. Record your activities each waking hour for the next 3 days.

3. Also write down when you have pain or feel fatigued.

4. After your log is completed, take three different colored highlighters and mark each hour of activity as low, moderate, or high energy. For example, you could use a yellow marker for low-energy activities, pink for moderate-energy, and green for high-energy.

5. Now analyze your log. Are your activities well balanced, or is there too much of one color? When are you feeling a lot of pain or especially fatigued? Which activities are really important to you, and which ones can you eliminate? What are you doing that is helping you to physically recover, and what is hindering your ability to mend?

It is interesting and helpful to see how your log "lights up." You may think you aren't doing much, but then you see that you have mostly pink and green in your log. Or vice versa. It doesn't really matter; the point is that it's a good place to start. You'll get a lot of valuable information from this exercise if you have the patience to do it.

Time Now and Time in the Future

When people are ill, they may be tempted to consider only the present. The future can seem uncertain in a way that it didn't before. Often well-intentioned doctors, family members, and friends urge people who are sick to "live in the present moment." I am not a big fan of using clichés with people who are ill or injured. Though I love words and how they go together, sometimes clichés can be a bit condescending and even disrespectful. Others in this genre include "Live for today"; "Today is the only day that counts"; and "Think about the here and now." The list is long and impressive.

Despite the overuse of such phrases, their message is relevant. They all boil down to the concept of mindfulness—full engagement in one's day-to-day life. This is an important topic, which I'll discuss in further detail in Chapter 9.

While concentrating on the here and now is valuable, as humans we are not able to completely avoid thinking about the future. Nor should we. As

Harvard psychologist Daniel Gilbert, PhD, notes, "The human being is the only animal that thinks about the future." Researchers studying this phenomenon, according to Dr. Gilbert, have found that about 12 percent of our daily thoughts are about the future. In his book *Stumbling on Happiness,* he shares with readers how we are all "part-time residents of tomorrow." He writes, "A permanent present—what a haunting phrase. How bizarre and surreal it must be to serve a life sentence in the prison of the moment, trapped forever in the perpetual now, a world without end, a time without later."

Why are humans the one species that considers the future? Why are we the only part-time residents of that uncharted territory? As Dr. Gilbert explains:

> The surprisingly right answer is that people find it gratifying to exercise control—not just for the futures it buys them, but for the exercise itself. Being effective—changing things, influencing things, making things happen—is one of the fundamental needs with which human brains seem to be naturally endowed, and much of our behavior from infancy onward is simply an expression of this penchant for control. . . . The fact is that human beings come into the world with a passion for control, they go out of the world the same way, and research suggests that if they lose their ability to control things at any point between their entrance and their exit, they become unhappy, helpless, hopeless, and depressed.

For some, thinking about the future may bring comfort and hope. For others, it may be full of unsettling or even terrifying emotions such as worry, fear, and uncertainty.

Spiritual writer Thomas Moore knows a lot about the worry that comes with an altered future. In *Dark Nights of the Soul: A Guide to Finding Your Way Through Life's Ordeals,* he writes:

> It is a mistake to think of illness only as an affliction of the body. . . . Serious illness is often a dark night of the soul. . . . Give yourself what you need at the deepest level. Care rather than cure. Organize your life to support the process. You are incubating your soul, not living a heroic adventure. Arrange life accordingly. Tone it down. Get what comforts you can, but don't move against the process.

Taking some time to consider the future and plan your goals is extraordinarily helpful when it comes to physical healing. In 2006, a consortium of organizations involved in the field of oncology care issued a report titled "From Cancer Patient to Cancer Survivor: Lost in Transition." The report highlighted how cancer survivors often become lost in the medical system after their acute treatment ends. One of the main recommendations to come out of the report was for health care providers to develop a "survivorship plan" for people who are finishing treatment.

Because I founded an oncology rehabilitation program called RESTORE that focuses on physical healing after cancer treatment, I have been asked to consult with numerous hospital administrators who are trying to address the needs that the report identified. In one instance, the person who was drafting a proposal for a survivorship center at an out-of-state hospital was an attorney and a cancer survivor. He e-mailed me the proposal along with a note that said something along the lines of "I don't think we need a formal plan for survivors; just offering medical services that go beyond acute cancer care is enough." I disagreed. I think that all survivors of serious injury and illness need a very specific plan in order to optimally recover. Such a plan helps take people from "survivorship" to "thrivorship." It requires someone to think about the future and helps to achieve optimal healing.

Regardless of whether thinking about the future inspires you or causes you angst, at this point it's important to take some time to make a plan and to work on your goals. After all, do you remember the story of Pandora? According to Greek mythology, Pandora was the first woman on earth. The gods endowed her with many talents and virtues—hence her name Pandora, meaning "all-gifted." Pandora had a box that she was instructed not to open, but alas, curiosity got the better of her. When she opened the box, the evil contained within spread throughout the world. Pandora hastened to close the lid, but the entire contents had escaped, except for one thing that lay at the bottom: hope.

Whenever I hear someone talk about "opening Pandora's box," I imagine a whirlwind of terror and chaos swirling out of the box, leaving behind the most precious gift of all—safe and forever present. There is hope in nearly every situation. It is what helps sustain us through our journey in the Healing Zone.

Make Time for a New Beginning

Virginia Woolf once wrote an essay on being ill in which she elegantly described what many others have experienced—that illness, with all its inherent problems and changes, also provides opportunities. Woolf said it this way: "Considering how common illness is, how tremendous the spiritual changes that it brings, how astonishing, when the light of health go down, the undiscovered countries that are then disclosed. . . . "

While no doubt there are "undiscovered countries" to explore, it doesn't mean that illness bestows "gifts" (though some people think so, that was not my experience). I don't like to think of illness as something that bears gifts; I worry that this concept is overly simplified and may marginalize people and their profound experiences. However, it is a fact that all of our experiences provide opportunities.

Being seriously ill changes your life. It takes you down an alternate path and shows you places that are different from what you've seen before. Almost always this path is dark and frightening. Always it is lonely, for the ill person ultimately travels alone.

As the darkness lifts and you enter the Healing Zone, there is opportunity and hope—a new beginning. It isn't a chance to go back to the person you were before, as that's not possible. Instead, this new beginning allows you to become the person you will be in the future—one who must incorporate your experience into the fabric of your life.

Sometimes it's helpful to recognize this new beginning for what it is—a turning point, a chance, a lifting of the "darkness." In *To Begin Again,* writer Naomi Levy provides an eloquent description of this transition.

> As the darkness lifts, don't let that moment pass without experiencing its full force. Talk a walk, even if it's only around the block. Breathe deeply. Gaze at the trees, listen to the birds, look up at the sky, take in the beauty. Eat your favorite food. Savor every bite with a renewed appetite for living. . . . Stand before a mirror and stare into your own eyes. See the hope that shines through. Tell yourself how far you have come and acknowledge the strength you never knew you had. Sit in a quiet place and talk to God. Express your full range of emotions. Your anger, frustration, and sadness, as well as your joy, relief, and optimism. Give thanks for the power to endure and carry on, for the new day and its promise, for all the blessings you have taken for granted.
>
> Then brace yourself for the struggles that are yet to come.

Taking the time to heal is an investment in you, your family, and your future. It is the most valuable gift you can give yourself and your loved ones.

Jeff Card

I'm 42 years old, and ever since age 17, I've had a recurring problem with deep vein thrombophlebitis, which is nothing more than blood clots developing in the calf of my right leg. The last episode, which happened in November 2005, also was the first I'd had in about 10 years. I was treated in the hospital for a week or so, and the clot went away. I was sent home on my regular oral blood thinner as well as a new injectable blood thinner.

It turns out that I had a bad reaction to the combination of the two anticoagulants. I started to bleed internally. I actually had a large bleed into the right side of my pelvis, which formed a relatively large hematoma [collection of blood] about the size of an avocado. This crushed the femoral nerve in my leg. I thought I just had another blood clot, and pain is pain—except this was much more excruciating at the time that it happened, and then it just kind of went away. But when it went away, so did all the feeling in my right leg. About a month after being released from the hospital, I realized the sensation was not coming back at all, and I had lost the use of my right leg.

At work, I'm a mergers-and-acquisitions specialist, so I travel an inordinate amount of time. I was in Southeast Asia a month before this happened, in Finland the week it happened, in New York the day it happened. Though I'm constantly traveling, I'm also constantly aware of the fact that I have this condition. I'm on blood thinner, and I'm smart enough to get up and walk around on planes and take care of myself. It just got the best of me this time.

I just wanted to get better. Here I'm at the top of my career, and I have a hundred people back at the office who are counting on me, and clients and kids and family, and I couldn't believe that this had happened. I thought that based upon previous experience, I'd be in the hospital for a week, home for a week, and then back to the office. Here it was going on a month. I remember the day I left the hospital, I was like, "Well, at least I'm out of the hospital. I just have to figure out how to get back."

It wasn't until a couple of weeks later, when I just was not getting any more movement in my leg, that I knew that I was in trouble. I was using crutches, using a walker, using my wife. Actually, pretty much when I came home from the hospital, I somehow made my way upstairs with the help of family and neighbors and never went downstairs for the first 2 weeks after that.

I have three school-age kids, and I went from a career where it was out of control in traveling away from home to all of a sudden being at home all the time. My children saw me during this time as someone other than who they were used to seeing. So it was very difficult for them. It was incredibly difficult for my wife, who just rose above it all to take care of the kids and make sure that they're okay and to make sure that I'm okay. It clearly frightens my wife and it frightens my kids—they just don't know what to expect. No one wants to see his or her partner or his or her father half the guy that he usually is. It's difficult.

When it happened, I asked that people respect my privacy and just let me get through it. At that point, I thought it would be something I'd get over quickly. But obviously, when you're gone from work for 4 months, people start to wonder and get concerned. So definitely they treat me differently. Since I've been back at work, I'm working full-time, but I work a lot from home. I still don't have my walk back; I walk with a cane. It's still very painful, although I try to hide it as much as possible. I think sometimes you just lose that battle and people see right through it.

I think you have to do a couple of things. First, you just have to dig down deep and don't settle for what physicians and doctors and caregivers are saying. Second, find help and don't be shy about it. I'm very fortunate in that I have the resources to do what I need to do, but you have to believe and know that if you don't have the resources, the help is still out there. Don't stop until you're satisfied with someone you've found who can help you.

It's a slow road to recovery, but what's comforting is the fact that now I understand what road I am on and there's a map. The map isn't 100 percent accurate, but it's pretty close. I can see that my body has responded a lot to the therapy, and I see myself hopefully regaining 100 percent of the use of my leg, if not pretty darn close to it, and getting back to the things that I like to do.

I believe that the human body is remarkable. All of a sudden you see an MRI of this big, huge avocado sitting in a fairly cramped space, knowing that it shouldn't be there, and then just trusting yourself, trusting your body will take care of it by absorbing it, and your nerve will somehow repair itself, and that you can, with the aid of therapists and doctors, get yourself back to normal. It just confirms the miracle that we are.

PART 2

Your Super Healing Plan

Chapter 5

Exercise to Build Strength and Endurance

Exercise is one of the three most important components of your Super Healing Plan. In fact, if there were a chemical formula for exercise that could be packaged as a pill, there is no doubt that it would be the most popular prescription drug available.

In the Super Healing Plan, I suggest that you make exercise a formal part of your day. Later on, I'll talk about the reasons for this. For now, just know that a structured program that includes setting goals and keeping track of certain parameters—such as the intensity and duration of an activity—will help you to heal faster and better.

Although many people can Super Heal at home, without a formal physical therapy prescription, it helps to know how medical doctors prescribe exercise. In a rehabilitation center, the physical and occupational therapists receive a written exercise prescription from a physician and then work with the patient on a therapeutic exercise program (what we often call Ther-Ex for short). This program is very specific and involves elements of the five main types of exercise training.

1. Aerobic (also called cardiovascular or endurance) exercises

2. Strengthening exercises

3. Flexibility (also called range of motion or stretching) exercises

4. Functional (also called coordination or balance training) exercises

5. Sport-specific exercises

In physical healing, the first two types—aerobic and strengthening— usually are the most important, though the others may need to be addressed, depending on your specific illness or injury and whether or not you are an athlete. These two categories of exercise offer multiple benefits, including:

- Enhancing immune system function
- Increasing blood volume and improving hemostasis
- Building strength
- Lowering cholesterol levels
- Strengthening bones
- Increasing lean body mass and helping to control weight
- Improving metabolism
- Helping to control blood sugar levels
- Promoting better balance and coordination
- Improving heart and lung function
- Reducing the risk of serious heart problems
- Promoting a positive outlook
- Reducing stress, anxiety, and depression
- Relieving fatigue
- Contributing to better sleep
- Reducing effort to perform work and home activities
- Fostering a sense of well-being
- Improving quality of life

Flexibility exercises may become important in a variety of situations. For example, after someone has a mastectomy for breast cancer, she (or he) may develop shoulder problems that improve with flexibility exercises. People with low back pain may need to work on hamstring flexibility to reduce spinal stress. As for functional exercises, they may be beneficial when, say, someone is experiencing balance and coordination issues after a stroke. For athletes, sport-specific training (e.g., running sprints, shooting baskets, or serving a tennis ball) is essential for optimal recovery.

These are just a few examples of how flexibility, functional, and sport-specific exercises can play a role in healing. In general, however, I recommend that most of the time you allot for exercise be spent on the first two categories, as they can have the greatest impact on physical recovery.

Therapeutic Exercise Is Essential

In Tolstoy's classic tale *Anna Karenina*, Konstantin Levin keeps himself strong and healthy by tending to his immense farm, even taking up a scythe to mow his fields. If you are a modern-day Levin who, in part, gets your exercise from mowing the lawn, will this help you to heal well? Not really.

First of all, how long you engage in this physical activity depends a lot on the size of your lawn. If it's small and you want to really get your heart rate up, do you then go and mow the neighbor's lawn? If it's a big lawn, do you mow part of it on one day and finish another day? The intensity of your workout will also depend on how high the grass is and what kind of mower you have. Neither of these parameters are ones that you can control very well, nor do they ensure an optimal workout. Then there is the problem of unintended breaks when you run out of gas or nature calls. Do you keep going to maintain your elevated heart rate by pushing a mower that is not cutting grass—or by wetting your pants?

Believe it or not, the question of exactly what constitutes exercise has been debated for thousands of years. Galen, physician to the gladiators and to Roman emperor Marcus Aurelius and his son Commodus, answered this question in the second century AD. He wrote, "To me it does not seem that all movement is exercise, but only when it is vigorous." A modern dictionary definition of exercise goes something like this: "bodily exertion for the sake of developing or maintaining physical fitness." So what counts as exercise? Does vacuuming? What about taking the stairs instead of the elevator? How about lifting bags of groceries or heavy boxes?

In the scientific literature, there is much discussion about "physical activity" versus "exercise" and whether all physical activity (e.g., mowing the lawn, vacuuming, walking to the mailbox) qualifies as exercise. Rather than enter that debate, what I want to emphasize here are the kinds of physical movement that facilitate optimal recovery. For example, if you are running around doing a lot of errands and chores, this is more likely to leave you fatigued than to promote healing. On the other hand, if you spent your time and energy on a more structured exercise program, you'd likely get greater therapeutic benefit. What it boils down to is, what are the best ways to exercise to facilitate healing and avoid excessive fatigue?

There is no doubt that physical activity is great for people, but a formal therapeutic exercise program will provide better results in less time—which means that in order to heal optimally, you would be better off asking someone else to cut your lawn so that you can focus your time and energy on exercises that will facilitate your recovery. While you are in the Healing Zone, if you are able to enlist someone else to perform physically draining rather than sustaining chores, give yourself permission to opt out of these activities.

Before we get into the details of how to set Super Healing exercise goals, I want to explain how physical activity can help you heal faster and better and perhaps even improve your prognosis.

How Exercise Can Help You Heal Better

Everyone knows that exercise helps keep people healthy, but how does it work to help us heal when we are seriously ill or injured?

Ironically, wars have given us the opportunity to explore things such as how exercise affects recovery. Though war undoubtedly is tragic, we have learned a lot about healing from every single major military endeavor, in large part because of the sheer number of injured subjects to study.

In the introduction, I described how the specialty of physical medicine and rehabilitation got its start in World War II because of the great need to rehabilitate the more than 600,000 injured military personnel. Years later, we learned something important about exercise and physical healing from the Vietnam War. At the time, military doctors noticed that soldiers with serious wounds who were evacuated stateside had delayed healing. Two military physicians, C. Robert Valeri, MD, and Mark D. Altschule, MD, published a paper on this phenomenon that they called the "missing blood syndrome." They correctly hypothesized that there was a "hidden" loss of blood volume in the injured soldiers, which contributed to the delayed healing. Blood transfusions seemed to "refill the limbs" and hasten recovery.

Later, in specific cases (including cancer and AIDS), doctors began to use a treatment that helped to increase the number of red blood cells (erythrocytes) in the blood. This therapy, rhEPO, is what is known as "blood doping" in sports. Its use by athletes is prohibited.

Since this is a chapter on the benefits of exercise in healing, you may be wondering what blood volume has to do with it. The exact mechanisms by which exercise accelerates wound healing are not known, but increasing blood volume is probably one of them. Increasing blood volume means that the oxygen and immune compounds that travel through the vascular system are more readily available to the tissues and organs that need them.

But it is not just blood volume that is a factor in exercise and healing. Exercise has a positive effect on hemostasis, which literally translated means "the stoppage of bleeding or hemorrhage." When we refer to hemostasis in medicine, what we often are discussing is the relationship of the chemical reactions in the blood—how they work together and influence each other.

For instance, exercise affects both aspects of the blood clotting system by simultaneously activating coagulation, which promotes blood clotting, and enhancing fibrinolysis, which has the opposite effect. When there is an imbalance in hemostasis in favor of too much coagulation, it leads to dangerous blood clots. If the imbalance is in favor of fibrinolysis, it can cause a life-threatening hemorrhage. So hemostasis involves a very complicated set of interactions, only two of which I've described here. What we know about exercise and hemostasis is that in the vast majority of people, physical activity improves the many variables involved in the process, and the net result is very positive.

Exercise also has a positive effect on the healing of muscles, bones, tendons, and ligaments. For example, the formation, or synthesis, of collagen helps injured tissues such as tendons to heal. You might think of collagen as the bricks that support many of our body's structures. Collagen synthesis is very important in healing, especially after surgery or trauma. In a study that assessed how exercise affected the collagen in a muscle and tendon at the knee, researchers found that "there is a rapid increase in collagen synthesis after strenuous exercise in human tendon and muscle."

Another way in which exercise may promote healing is by reducing excessive scar tissue, called fibrosis. In one study, excessive scar tissue declined by 50 percent with exercise.

How Exercise Can Help You Heal Faster

All of the above are examples of how exercise can help us to heal better, which is extremely important if we want to recapture our former strength and vitality. But exercise also helps us to heal faster.

The study that identified an increase in collagen production after exercise strongly suggests that this is a factor in how exercise helps us to heal better and faster. In another study evaluating the effects of exercise on wound healing, researchers assessed an initial group of 28 sedentary older adults who were known to be in good health. It was hypothesized that a 3-month program of aerobic exercise would significantly enhance wound healing. The participants were separated into two groups—a control group that remained sedentary and an exercise group. Each person in the study underwent a procedure that involved making a small wound in the skin of the upper arm. The wounds were the same size and depth, and the researchers measured them at regular intervals.

The results made headline news when they revealed that exercise indeed had a significant impact on wound healing. It took an average of 29 days for the exercisers' wounds to heal; in the control group, the average was 40 days. The study, the first of its kind, was published in 2005 in the *Journal of Gerontology*. More research is needed on how exercise can accelerate wound healing, but these are very exciting preliminary findings.

In the same study, the researchers measured cortisol levels in the saliva of the participants. Prolonged high cortisol levels, which are associated with stress, tend to slow healing. Physical stress such as exercise temporarily raises cortisol levels. It is believed to be the regulation of cortisol by the body—the ability to release it appropriately rather than at persistently high levels—that enhances immune function. The scientists who conducted the study concluded that exercise significantly enhanced wound healing. Though they are not sure of how this works, they suggested two logical explanations.

1. Exercise was shown to enhance immune function, and this may be related to how cortisol and other chemicals are released when we are physically active.

2. Exercise accelerates and enhances blood flow. As the scientists surmised, "Exercise may contribute to blood flow to the skin and increased skin oxygen tension, thereby enhancing wound-healing rates."

How Exercise Might Improve Your Prognosis

Research also suggests that with many conditions, the overall prognosis improves with regular physical activity. This means that exercise supports healing *and* helps prevent further medical problems in the future.

For example, most people know that there is a very strong link between exercise and preventing a heart attack or stroke. However, many people don't realize that exercise helps reduce the risk of contracting many other illnesses, including cancer. In medical terms, this means that exercise helps reduce the risk of a primary malignancy (a first or initial cancer).

This is important information for people to have, and it should be in a book on preventive health care. But this is a book on physical healing—filled with tips about what happens after you've already crossed into the Healing Zone. So the question that is paramount for those who have already been diagnosed with cancer is, can exercise help prevent their cancer from returning?

This is an exciting area of oncology research, and the preliminary answer seems to be a qualified yes. It's qualified because the research is at a very early stage, and while the initial results are quite positive for some cancers (breast and colon in particular), it's far too early to determine how effective exercise will be in preventing recurrence and which types of cancer will most benefit.

Heart disease, stroke, and cancer are the top three serious medical conditions that people in developed countries are likely to encounter. Exercise is exceedingly important in all of them in terms of physical recovery and the possibility of an improved prognosis. Moreover, exercise may improve the prognosis for other conditions, including chronic diseases such as fibromyalgia, arthritis, osteoporosis, and low back pain. In the majority of chronic conditions, those affected who exercise regularly and appropriately tend to have a better prognosis and experience less pain and disability.

So exercise helps you to heal faster and better, and it may improve your overall prognosis. Though the research on how exercise facilitates physical healing is evolving, and we still don't understand all of the reasons that exercise is such a potent therapy, we do know that it is a powerful method of encouraging optimal healing. Of course, it makes sense that when you are sick, you become weaker and have less strength and endurance.

As you may recall from Chapter 1, the rate of muscular decline with inactivity can be as high as 1 to 3 percent per day. After 3 or more weeks, it's possible to lose as much as 50 percent of your muscle strength. But as you can see from the research on exercise and healing, there is much more to this equation than simply regaining strength. Exercise has many profound and wonderful outcomes when it comes to physical recovery—which is why it is one of the three most important factors in Super Healing.

Getting Started

Several reputable organizations, including the American Heart Association and the American College of Sports Medicine, offer formal exercise guidelines that include information on when to perform tests (such as a cardiac stress test) prior to beginning an exercise program. These guidelines are very useful, but they do not address what to do if you are recovering from a serious injury or illness. I encourage everyone to check in with his or her "conductor" (physician) about how to safely exercise. The discussion should include what types of activities you can do, how hard you can push yourself, what you should avoid, and what problems you may encounter and should watch out for.

In the Super Healing Plan, you will start with one short-term and one long-term exercise goal. Prior to setting goals, it's fun and easy to test your current physical status, so you have some idea of what would be reasonable goals for you. On pages 68 and 69, there are several tests that you can do now and repeat later to measure your progress. Page 72 offers some suggestions about exercise goals, but be sure to review your goals with your physician.

If you have had surgery, your doctor likely will not want you to exercise within a month or so of the operation. Of course, the type of surgery makes a difference. For example, removing a gallbladder with tiny incisions through a laparoscope is very different from open-heart surgery, which involves a big incision and opening the chest and bony sternum. You also

(continued on page 70)

Baseline Walking Tests

The following three walking tests can help determine your walking baseline. You don't need to do more than one walk (or run) test. The point is to gather data to help you create goals and progress appropriately. You can repeat the test once a month to adjust your goals—or just for fun to see how you are improving.

Counting steps: Buy a pedometer and count your steps for 1 week. Then take your average daily count and try to increase it by 10 percent per week. So if you are currently walking an average of 2,000 steps per day, then your goal for next week would be 2,200 steps per day, and your short-term goal for the month would be 2,800 steps per day. You might advance a little slower or faster, which is fine. The 10 percent per week is just a guideline.

I usually advise people to set an initial long-term goal of 5,000 steps per day and then a second goal of 10,000 steps per day. You may reach your long-term goals before the 6-month point, depending on what level you start at and how quickly you advance.

1-, or 6-, or 12-minute walk (or run) test: For this test, you simply measure how far you can walk (or run) in 1, 6, or 12 minutes. If you are able to walk for 12 minutes, use that as your time frame. If that's uncomfortable, go with either the 1-minute or 6-minute time frame. You can do the test on a track, where you know the distance around the perimeter, or walk or run around your neighborhood and then drive the same route to check the mileage on your odometer. Also, take your pulse for 1 minute at the beginning of your walk or run and again at the end, and record this information.

An initial short-term goal would be to increase how far you are able to go in the allotted time by 10 percent over the course of a month. For example, if you covered 1 mile in the 12-minute walk test, then your short-term goal would be to walk 1.1 miles in 12 minutes.

Rockport 1-Mile Walk Test: This is a variation on the 6- or 12-minute walk test. What you do is check your heart rate before and after a 1-mile walk. Time yourself during the walk, then record your heart rate and your time in your log. As an initial short-term goal, you could aim to improve your time by 10 percent over the course of the month. So if you cover the mile in 15 minutes, next month's goal would be to go the same distance in 13.5 minutes—cutting your time by 1.5 minutes.

Baseline Strength Tests

These two tests are simple to perform. You can do just one or try both of them. Once you have a strength-training baseline, you'll be better able to define appropriate strength-training goals. Repeat these tests once a month to measure your progress. (*Note:* Please remember to check with your doctor before you begin a strength-training program.)

Pushup test: This test is done by counting how many pushups you can do without taking a break. You can perform the pushups either with your legs straight or with your knees bent and resting on the floor. Either way, keep your back straight and avoid touching your belly to the floor as you descend. Your hands should be shoulder-width apart, and you should lower yourself until your chin barely touches the ground.

Again, a reasonable short-term goal is to increase the number of pushups you can do by 10 percent over the course of a month. So if you can do 20 pushups now, then set a short-term goal of 22.

Situp test: For this test, you will need masking tape and a metronome. To set up the test, lie on your back on a flat surface with your knees bent at 90-degree angles and your arms straight against your sides, palms facing down. Place a piece of masking tape at the tips of your fingers on each side. (It's easier if someone helps you do this.) Next, measure 4 inches in front of each piece of tape. Place another piece of tape at this point on each side.

Set the metronome at 50 beats per minute. While lying on your back, slowly curl forward until your fingers reach the second set of taped lines. Do as many situps as you can in 1 minute without pausing. If you complete the test, you'll have done a total of 25.

You can set a number of different goals with this test, depending on how well you do as a baseline. For example, if you can manage only 10 situps, then your first short-term goal can be to increase by 5 over the course of a month. If you can squeeze out 25, you might decide to keep going and see how many more you can do. Let's say you complete 30 without stopping. Next month, you might aim for 40, using the metronome to keep time. You also can do this without the metronome, simply counting how many situps you can do in 1 minute.

will want to talk with your doctor about any symptoms you are having, especially postoperative pain, as it may affect your ability to exercise.

In general, you should skip or avoid exercise if you:

- Recently had surgery and haven't been cleared by your doctor
- Have any type of infection, including a wound infection or an upper respiratory infection
- Have uncontrolled pain, nausea, or other treatment side effects
- Feel dizzy or unstable and haven't been cleared by your doctor to exercise with these symptoms
- Have a fever higher than 100°F
- Had chemotherapy within the past 24 hours (check with your doctor about when to exercise following chemotherapy or other treatments)
- Have low blood cell counts (it's up to your doctor to determine safe levels)

Stop exercising immediately if you experience:

- Excessive fatigue or shortness of breath
- Heart palpitations
- Chest, jaw, or arm pain
- Dizziness or light-headedness

Report any of these symptoms to your doctor.

Also, before you begin your exercise program, it's a good idea to figure out what your target heart rate should be during aerobic exercise (see page 74). A doctor might opt for formal testing such as an electrocardiogram (EKG) or a cardiac stress test (usually done on a treadmill or with an upper extremity bike). She also may suggest physical or occupational therapy, particularly if a patient is very debilitated or has other medical issues such as postoperative musculoskeletal pain, delayed wound healing or scarring, or underlying health problems such as diabetes or heart disease. At my center, we often perform formal exercise testing to see what people are able to tolerate under supervised conditions. This includes monitoring vital signs such as blood pressure, heart rate, respiratory rate, and blood oxygen level (by using a pulse oximeter that clips onto a person's finger).

How to Make Exercise Fun and Stay Motivated

As you begin, you will find that exercise is much easier if you make it a habit—something that you do regularly without giving it much thought.

This is important when you're using physical activity to heal optimally. Establishing a new habit takes concentration and planning, but once you have it down, it becomes just as second nature as brushing your teeth or putting on your seat belt when you get in your car.

Everyone who exercises gets bored at some point. Let's face it—physical activity is work. Sometimes work is challenging and fun; other times it's tedious and frustrating. This is true of exercise, no matter what your skill level is or how much you've done in the past. Nevertheless, there are things that you can do to help maintain your motivation to exercise. For example:

Consider your personality. What do you like to do? Let's say you begin your exercise regimen with walking (which is a great starter activity, as I explain in the next section). If you like solitude, you might find a nature trail. If you like action, walk in a busy park. Perhaps you are an indoor kind of person; then walk in a mall or on a treadmill. Maybe you like variety, so each day you'll go to a different place. Whatever you choose is fine. Just think about what you'll enjoy the most.

Include others. You can ask a family member or friend to accompany you on your activity (e.g., riding bike or swimming together). Joining a class or club is another way to get out and interact with others.

Vary your routine. The more you vary your exercise, the more engaging it will be. Athletes refer to this as cross-training. Doing a lot of different kinds of exercise is a great way to stay motivated, and it's really good for your body. I'll explain more about cross-training later in the chapter.

Have fun. Consider doing things that you haven't done in ages. When was the last time you went dancing or skating? Make plans to rent a rowboat or canoe and enjoy an afternoon on the water. Snowshoe or hike in the woods. Adding music to any activity can make it more enjoyable. Likewise, using an exercise gadget such as a pedometer or heart rate monitor can add an element of variety and fun to your routine.

Be flexible. Suppose you planned to walk in the park today, but it's raining. Not a problem; just go to the mall instead. Or what if you had planned to exercise this morning, but you woke up with a terrible headache? No need to fret. Instead, try to treat your headache, and then exercise later in the day—or just skip it altogether.

Take a break when you need to. If you need to take a day, a week, or even a month off from your exercise program, don't feel guilty about it. Guilt leads to stress, and stress isn't good for your body or spirit. Instead, plan a time when you can get back on track, and congratulate yourself for doing so.

Reward yourself. Consider setting up a reward system for yourself as you accomplish your exercise goals. Actually, you can reward yourself just

Short- and Long-Term Exercise Goals

I offer these short- and long-term goals as examples for when you set your own. They aren't meant to be the ones that you adopt for yourself; rather, use them as a jumping-off point.

As you write your goals, don't worry about whether they are perfect. Chances are they won't be, and you'll need to adjust them later on. That's a normal part of the process. I encourage you to simply write your goals, and then reevaluate them in a month's time.

Short-Term (Aerobic)

1. Obtain a pedometer and keep a log of how many steps you are taking on a daily basis. Then increase this number by 10 percent, or by 500 to 1,000 steps a day.
2. Take a daily walk around a track, in your neighborhood, or at the mall.
3. Join a water aerobics class.
4. Make a habit of using your stationary bicycle, stairclimber, or elliptical trainer whenever you talk on the phone. Keep track of the minutes.

Short-Term (Strengthening)

1. Perform the pushup test and use this as your baseline. Increase the number of pushups that you can do by 10 percent.
2. Perform the situp test and use this as your baseline. Increase the number of situps that you can do by 10 percent.
3. Begin your strength-training program with the three exercises described on page 78. Increase gradually—usually 10 percent every 4 weeks is reasonable.
4. Make an appointment with a physical therapist or a personal trainer to develop an appropriate exercise program for you.

Long-Term Goals

1. Perform one of the walking tests described on page 68. Try to improve your score by 25 to 50 percent over the course of 6 months.
2. Consistently do some form of aerobic exercise almost every day.
3. Consistently do strengthening exercises 2 or 3 days a week.
4. Check in regularly with your personal trainer or physical therapist over the course of 6 months to advance your exercise program.

for participating in physical activity, regardless of whether you meet your goals. Taking time to acknowledge your accomplishments can go a long way toward maintaining your motivation.

Begin with Walking

As previously mentioned, walking is a great way to ease into an exercise program—one that has been prescribed since ancient times. Around 400 BC, Hippocrates wrote a book on preventive medicine called *Regimen in Health* in which he advocated walking slowly in the summer and quickly during winter months. Over time, walking has become perhaps the most popular form of physical activity. One reason is that almost everyone can do it. (If you can't walk, you might try an activity that limits or doesn't involve leg use, such as swimming, water aerobics, or upper-extremity cycling or rowing. Ask your doctor about what else might be safe to try.)

In his book *Flow: The Psychology of Optimal Experience,* Mihaly Csikszentmihalyi describes how walking, a seemingly simple task, offers much in the way of setting goals and achieving them. He comments:

> Walking is the most trivial physical activity imaginable, yet it can be profoundly enjoyable if a person sets goals and takes control of the process. . . . A great number of different goals might be set for a walk. For instance, the choice of the itinerary: where one wishes to go, and by what route. Within the overall route, one might select places to stop, or certain landmarks to see. Another goal may be to develop a personal style, a way to move the body easily and efficiently. An economy of motion that maximizes physical well-being is another obvious goal. For measuring progress, the feedback may include how fast and how easily the intended distance was covered; how many interesting sights one has seen; and how many new ideas or feelings were entertained along the way.

In 2002, snowboarder Chris Klug won a bronze medal at the Winter Olympics. Eighteen months prior to his incredible victory, Klug had undergone a lifesaving liver transplant because of a condition called primary sclerosing cholangitis, which earlier had claimed the life of football great Walter Payton. What is remarkable about Klug is not only his amazing athletic prowess but also his dedication to healing optimally. When I talked with Klug, he told me that the first thing he did after his surgery was to walk around the hospital. After he was discharged, he began a more intense walking program that included touring the city of Denver, where he was temporarily staying to be close to his doctors. Though Csikszentmihalyi describes walking as "the most trivial physical activity imaginable," it is a relatively complex process that helps to improve balance, strength, and endurance throughout the body.

I recommend investing in a pedometer so you can record how many steps you take over the course of a day. At first, all you are doing is figuring

Target Heart Rate

It's a good idea to try to keep within your target heart rate (THR) range during aerobic activities. When you're just starting to exercise, you may want to stay toward the lower end of the range. As you get stronger and build endurance, you can push yourself a bit harder, toward the upper end of your range. Record your range in your exercise log, so you can easily refer to it.

You can monitor your heart rate by taking your pulse at your wrist or your neck. Another inexpensive option is to purchase a heart rate monitor. You can find these in sporting goods stores and at many online retailers.

In someone who hasn't been training, resting heart rate usually is between 60 and 100 beats per minute. A young adult has a maximum heart rate (MHR) between 190 and 200, while for a middle-aged and older adult, MHR is between 140 and 160.

If you already have done some exercise testing, you may have been told your THR or THR range. Otherwise, you can calculate them yourself with these simple formulas.

$$MHR = 220 - your age$$
$$THR (lower limit) = 0.6 \times MHR$$
$$THR (upper limit) = 0.8 \times MHR$$

Let's say you're 40 years old. Your MHR is 180 (220 − 40 = 180). This means the lower limit of your THR range is 108 (0.6 × 180), while the upper limit is 144 (0.8 × 180). You can round off these numbers and use 110 to 150 as your THR range, which means that you try to raise your heart rate above 110 but not higher than 150. THR goals can be a bit higher for people who are very fit and a bit lower for people who have heart conditions or are on blood pressure medication.

out how active you are during the day. With this as your baseline, you can set a short-term and long-term goal that involves increasing the number of steps you are taking. Usually a reasonable initial short-term goal is to increase your average number of steps by 500 to 1,000 per day (or use the 10 percent rule). The goal for active, healthy people is 10,000 steps per day, so consider this number when you are creating your long-term goal. Ten thousand steps per day may not be realistic for everyone; I offer this simply as an example of a good benchmark for people without any health restrictions.

Most people enjoy wearing a pedometer; many of my patients tell me that it is the single best piece of advice that I have given them. On page 68, I also describe several tests that you can perform to establish your walking baseline. All of the tests are fun to do, and you can set your exercise goals based on the results of the test you choose. In addition, it's encouraging to retake the test at a 4-week interval and note your progress.

Utilize Cross-Training for Maximum Benefit

Cross-training involves alternating the activities in your exercise routine in order to maximize the benefits while reducing the risk of injury. For example, swimming is a wonderful aerobic exercise, but it doesn't support bone health like a weight-bearing exercise such as walking does. Also, it is not uncommon for swimmers, especially those who don't cross-train, to end up with shoulder problems from overuse. Likewise, walking is a great aerobic exercise, but it works the lower body more than the upper body.

As you consider how best to cross-train, it's important to think about whether you want to do open- or closed-chain exercises or a mix of both types. In open-chain exercises such as walking, your feet break contact with the surface at some point. In a closed-chain exercise such as using an elliptical trainer, your feet remain on the surface at all times, which generates less force through your joints. Closed-chain kinetic exercises (e.g., cycling, stairclimbing, rowing) tend to be easier on your joints and back because you avoid the pounding that occurs with open chain-exercises (e.g., walking, running, skating).

Cross-training not only helps get your body in the best shape possible, it also helps make your exercise program a lot more interesting. So while I recommend starting with walking and keeping track of your steps, when you feel up to it, try adding some other types of aerobic exercise. Among your options:

- Hiking
- Jogging
- Tennis
- Basketball

- Rowing
- Cycling
- Roller- or ice-skating
- In-line skating
- Swimming
- Walking in water
- Treading water
- Water aerobics

- Soccer
- Dancing
- Jumping rope
- Aerobics
- Stairclimbing, elliptical, or spinning machine
- Cross-country skiing
- Snowshoeing

Add Strength Training to Your Regimen

During the 1800s, exercise was thought to be good for the spirit and to help build character. Some touted it as a moral obligation, giving rise to the phrase "muscular Christianity." While I wouldn't go so far as to say that strength training is a moral obligation, I will say that it can do a lot to help you to heal optimally. I do recommend checking with your doctor before starting or resuming a strength-training program.

Since I know that everyone has various levels of experience with strength training, and I want to keep things as uncomplicated as possible for your journey through the Healing Zone, I'll offer several suggestions for how to begin (or resume) a strengthening regimen. If you are able, I encourage you to perform at least one of the baseline strength tests described on page 69. Then consider these options and choose the one that best suits your experience and current physical condition.

1. If you have no previous training or are recovering from a very serious illness or injury, consider asking your doctor for a prescription to see a physical therapist. The prescription should say something like "Therapeutic exercise focusing on improving strength and cardiovascular fitness. Transition to home exercise program—provide strategies for this transition."

2. Consult a personal trainer. Though the credentialing process for trainers is quite inconsistent (which means that the quality of personal trainers can vary widely), finding a good trainer can be very helpful. You should look for someone who understands your health status and tailors your strength-training regimen accordingly rather than just telling you to "work harder." When my patients have problems after

working with a trainer, it almost always is because the trainer doesn't pay attention to the patient's health issues and has a "no pain, no gain" attitude. Seek out a trainer who is thoughtful and knowledgeable. For tips, see "How to Choose a Personal Trainer." Your doctor or physical therapist might be able to suggest a qualified trainer. You also can check out your local gym or ask someone who has used a trainer in the past for a referral. When you talk with a trainer, you'll get a good sense of whether this person is only interested in pushing you physically or is going to support your efforts to heal optimally.

How to Choose a Personal Trainer

Personal trainers vary widely in experience and qualifications. If you are considering using one, make sure that he or she meets the following professional and training criteria.

Choose someone certified. Though the certification requirements are not uniform nationally, you want to select a trainer who has gone through a formal certification process. The American Council on Exercise is the largest nonprofit certifying organization in the world.

Ask for references. It's really helpful to talk with a personal trainer's clients and get a sense of how enthusiastic they are about this fitness professional. Be sure to ask how the trainer handles health issues when they arise.

Review the trainer's business practices. Ideally, the person with whom you work will have policies and procedures in writing. This includes information about fees, billing, the cancellation policy, and liability insurance.

Insist on a trainer who understands your health needs. A good trainer will ask you to complete a health questionnaire and then review it with you. He or she will develop your exercise program to accommodate any medical issues that you may have.

Decide if this is someone you will feel comfortable working with. Are you pleased with the arrangements, including where you would meet, what time of day, and how many times each week?

Trust your gut. You have good instincts, so trust them. If you like the trainer and think that the two of you can work together, you likely will have a good relationship that will facilitate your physical recovery.

3. If you were following a strengthening routine before your illness or injury, then slowly ease back into it. You want your body to get accustomed to strength training again. Most people can safely advance by 10 percent (in resistance and repetitions) at each short-term-goal mark (4 weeks). You may feel able to progress more quickly, but it's always better to take a slow and steady approach than to do too much too soon, get injured, and then quit altogether.

What follows are three very basic strength-training exercises—one for your core (the middle of your body, which supports everything else), another for your arms, and the third for your legs. For most people, this sequence should be relatively easy to do.

Core: Take the situp test (see page 69). Increase by 10 percent, or 5 to 10 situps, over the course of 4 weeks. (Double this if you change your goal every 8 weeks, as described below.)

Arms: Take the pushup test (see page 69). Increase by 10 percent, or 5 to 10 pushups, every 4 weeks. (Double up if you're changing your goal every 8 weeks.)

Legs: Perform a modified squat by sitting down in a chair (with or without using your arms for support, depending on if you need to) and then rising. Repeat 10 to 15 times, followed by a 2-minute rest. Do the entire sequence again. You can also do this by standing with your back against a wall and sliding down, as though you were sitting in a chair, and then pushing back up with your legs.

Since these exercises don't cover all the muscle groups, it isn't a complete program. But when you're starting out, the most important thing is to avoid injury. My suggestion is to build your Super Healing goals around this sequence. You can always progress faster or slower.

For suggestions on short- and long-term exercise goals, refer to page 72. You might want to alternate your short-term goals between aerobic activity and strength training. For example, you could start with a short-term goal for aerobic exercise. You'll be working on this goal for 8 weeks, because at the 4-week mark, you'll add a short-term goal for strength training. At the next 4-week mark (8 weeks after your start date), you'll create a new goal for aerobic activity. Four weeks later, you'll create a new goal for strengthening, and so on. This way, you have just one new goal every 4 weeks, but you are working on improving both endurance and strength.

Ready, Set . . . Super Heal

Most people are well aware of the importance of exercise in promoting good health and preventing disease. Robert Levine, MD, writes, "The

Exercise Adaptations for Medical Problems

Most people can exercise safely, but it's important to consider how best to go about it. These are some suggestions for how you might want to modify your exercise regimen to accommodate specific medical issues.

Arthritis: Non-weight-bearing cardiovascular exercises such as cycling and swimming prevent stress on joints. Taking breaks is helpful to minimize pain. Strengthening muscles around painful joints can be achieved with isometric exercises, which involve no movement. Instead, you simply tighten the muscle—in your thigh, for example—and hold for 8 to 10 seconds. Open-chain exercise, in which the foot is not in contact with the ground or floor, is one way to work a lower extremity without adding stress to joints. For example, you could lie on your back and raise one foot about 6 inches off the floor. Hold for 30 seconds.

Diabetes: Aerobic activities may reduce blood sugar levels, so it is important to monitor this carefully. Lower load and higher repetitions are recommended for strengthening exercises. Be sure there is no chafing or breakdown of skin on your feet from sweating.

Back pain: Lumbar-stabilization exercises are recommended to improve core (middle of the body) muscle strength and flexibility. Generally, avoid high-load (e.g., heavy weight or strong resistance) strengthening exercises.

Osteoporosis: Weight-bearing exercises—both aerobic and muscle-strengthening—help to strengthen bones. Swimming and water aerobics, while good for your heart, don't help bones as much as other activities because they are non-weight-bearing.

Hypertension: Strengthening is best done with a lower load and higher repetitions, while avoiding isometric exercises (which involve a sustained muscular contraction rather than moving through a range). Monitor blood pressure or perceived exhaustion when performing aerobic exercises, and avoid holding your breath.

Limb limitations: Some people have limited use of their legs because of paralysis, injury, or surgery. In terms of cardiovascular exercise, here are some activities that limit or don't involve the legs.

- Swimming
- Water aerobics
- Chair aerobics
- Upper-extremity cycling
- Upper-extremity rowing
- Cardio punching bag
- Upper-extremity circuit training

evidence supporting the value of exercise in terms of reducing various diseases and overall mortality is overwhelming to the point that people who avoid physical activity do so at their own peril." What people generally are not as aware of is the incredible impact of exercise on physical healing. As you travel through the Healing Zone, if you want to recover faster and better—and potentially improve your overall prognosis—you'll need to add therapeutic exercise to your Super Healing Plan.

REMARKABLE RECOVERY

Chris Klug

I was in the 11th hour of the liver transplant waiting process. When I got to that 11th hour, I started to lose hope. I knew the realities of it. But at the same time, I kept pushing forward. I was on the transplant list for 6 years total and for 3 months at the critical stage. I couldn't even play golf; I was pretty wrecked. I would go to the gym and cheer my brother and my buddies on, thinking that maybe I got some benefit just by being there.

With a liver transplant, I pretty much got cut in half. I was in surgery for 6 hours, and the next day I was walking around the hospital. I had to carry my little IV tree. The doctor had to keep me on a pretty tight leash. I felt like a new engine got dropped in me. I just knew I was going to make it back. I also knew I had some serious damage to overcome. As a professional athlete, I have a short window to do what I love.

I was released from the hospital 4 days later. For the next 3 weeks, I stayed in a hotel in Denver. I walked everywhere. I just walked up and down in Denver's downtown. That seemed to really help me a lot. It got my blood flowing. I was able to exercise, but it didn't allow too much impact.

I went back on snow 7 weeks later, and I wasn't sure what would happen if I crashed. It was a little bit scary, but I wanted to get back to doing what I love. I remember getting back on snow, and visualization played a big role in that for me. I do a lot of visualization in sports. You have to see it to make it happen. As I sat in the hospital, I visualized what it would be like to snowboard again. It's all perspective and where you set the bar.

One and a half years after my transplant, I won the bronze medal in the Olympics. Even then things didn't go perfectly for me. When I won my bronze medal, I broke my boot and duct-taped it. I learned I had to make do.

I like to talk about my two great races—my snowboard race and my race for life.

Chapter 6

Eat to Heal Your Body

The second key factor in your ability to Super Heal has to do with how you fuel your tissues and organs. Food provides the necessary nutrients to help your body's one trillion cells recover. No matter what kind of injury or illness you are facing, what and how you eat will determine the course of your physical mending.

Benjamin Franklin had something to say about practically everything. One topic that he frequently spoke and wrote about was diet. While some of his ideas have not stood the test of time (for example, he extolled the virtues of nudity and made a point of spending a portion of his day in his birthday suit), his nutrition recommendations generally were quite sound. Recent scientific research has confirmed what many intellectuals such as Franklin have surmised for centuries—that what we eat has extremely important implications for health and disease. Among Franklin's dietary witticisms:

- To lengthen thy life, lessen thy meals.
- Three good [big] meals a day is bad living.
- Eat to live, and not live to eat.
- Many dishes, many diseases.

Franklin also summed up the folly of a poor diet combined with lack of exercise in this rather dramatic manner: "Nine men in ten are would-be suicides." It may seem like an outrageous statement, but the truth is that, genes aside, we do have some control over our health destinies through the choices we make every day, particularly regarding what we eat and how we exercise. These two lifestyle factors have the greatest impact on preventing and healing from serious illness.

The Diet Dilemma

Of course, popular culture—which is too often fueled by a sensationalistic media—has focused on dietary issues in a manner that has left many people both bewildered and anxious. Are we poisoning our bodies with what we eat? Must we adhere to an extreme dietary regimen to have a long, healthy life? Should our medicine cabinets be chock-full of supplements to make up for all of the nutrients missing from our diets?

There is no doubt that we need food to survive and we need food to heal. Unfortunately, the advice we're given about what we should (and should not) eat can be incredibly confusing and often contradictory. In a historical look at gluttony, one of the seven deadly sins, author Francine Prose writes, "Obviously, our culture exhibits a schizophrenic attitude toward gluttony. One minute, we're bombarded with images of food, advertisements for restaurants, or the latest sweet or fatty snack, with recipes and cooking tips. A minute later, we're reminded that eating is tantamount to suicide, that indulgence and enjoyment equals social isolations and self-destruction."

Indeed, literally thousands of books address diet and nutrition—many written by very reputable authors who don't necessarily offer similar advice. One physician-author whose insights are extremely thoughtful and reputable is Walter Willett, MD, chairman of the department of nutrition at Harvard Medical School. In 2001, Dr. Willett published the groundbreaking book *Eat, Drink, and Be Healthy,* in which he charged that the U.S. Department of Agriculture (USDA) dietary recommendations—taught to children in grade school in the form of the food pyramid—were wrong. In Dr. Willett's words: "At best, the USDA Pyramid offers wishy-washy, scientifically unfounded advice on an absolutely vital topic—what to eat. At worst, the misinformation contributes to overweight, poor health, and unnecessary early deaths."

Dr. Willett clearly was frustrated by the information that the general public has been getting about what to eat. He cites as an example the "Great Nutrition Debate," sponsored by the USDA in 2000, in which the authors of several best-selling diet books discussed their philosophies. Dr. Willett describes the event as a "mostly evidence-free food fight." He goes on to say, "The wildly different recommendations presented in that 3-hour session—eat lots of meat, don't eat any meat, eat lots of carbohydrates, don't eat any carbohydrates, cut your intake of fat to under 20 percent of calories, eat as much fat as you want, stay away from sugar, eat potatoes—neatly captured the chaos that we get in place of sound, sensible, and solid advice on healthy eating."

Following this debate, USDA undersecretary Shirley Watkins commented, "We will stand behind the pyramid." But Watkins was forced to eat her words (so to speak) in the wake of tremendous pressure—including from Dr. Willett's book—to revise the food pyramid to make it more representative of what we know scientifically about the parameters of a healthy diet. Hence, today we have a new USDA food pyramid that, though not perfect, is a marked improvement from what was widely taught just a few years ago.

Two medical doctors who have written quite a bit about what we should eat are cardiologist Dean Ornish, MD, and the late Robert Atkins, MD. Interestingly, these doctors are at opposite ends of the dietary spectrum, with Dr. Atkins proposing a low-carbohydrate, high-fat diet and Dr. Ornish stressing a low-fat vegetarian-type diet. With comments that pushed their two opposing dietary philosophies into the national spotlight, Dr. Ornish at one point charged Dr. Atkins with being "irresponsible" and accused him of trying to sell books by telling people to eat steak and eggs. Dr. Atkins responded by defending his diet and publicly questioning Dr. Ornish's credibility.

The very different approaches of these two doctors simply serve to highlight the fact that there continues to be tremendous controversy about what we should be eating. In this chapter, I'm going to focus on what to eat to heal your body optimally. This is something that is rarely discussed, even by leading experts on diet and nutrition, but it is extremely important.

In order to Super Heal, you need to consider how the food you eat will help your body repair cell damage. I will offer advice that is based on my undergraduate degree in food biochemistry, combined with my medical training and many years of experience in treating people who are seriously injured or ill. While some of my advice draws on scientific studies, because of large gaps in our knowledge about food and healing, I also will be making suggestions that at this time seem logical and appropriate for people who are in the Healing Zone.

As you read this chapter, keep in mind that I am not trying to debate the incredible amount of dietary information and misinformation available via media outlets and the Internet. Rather, I want to share with you what we know about how food supports the healing process.

One more thought before we go any further: Remember that the Bill Clinton "one wrong step" rule does not apply to diet. You can't eat one wrong food or even a bunch of junk food and anticipate disastrous results. Your body can handle quite a bit, and while paying attention to how you nourish it is important, worrying about every bite is not worthwhile or necessary.

How Food Heals

There is no doubt that what you eat can help you to heal. For example:

- Vitamin A supports skin and bone health and plays a role in immune function.

- Vitamin C, a tissue antioxidant, is necessary for collagen formation and immune function.

- Vitamin E is a potent antioxidant.

- Bromelain—a group of enzymes derived from the pineapple plant—reduces swelling, bruising, and pain and speeds healing time following trauma or surgery.

- Glucosamine is important for wound healing.

- Adequate protein is absolutely essential for optimal healing. Specific amino acids—the building blocks of protein—that appear to be especially critical to the healing process include arginine and glutamine.

- Zinc is necessary for DNA synthesis, protein synthesis, and cell growth.

This is a short and incomplete list. The point here is that food provides many, many incredibly important nutrients that assist with physical recovery.

It would be interesting—but unethical—to conduct a study in which people in need of physical healing are divided into two groups—one that receives a nutritious diet and the other that does not. There was similar research, actually, only it involved healthy national-level judo athletes. For this study, one group underwent significant food restriction, while the other group (the control group) didn't. The purpose of the research was to determine whether food restriction affected physical performance and levels of certain compounds in the body.

At the end of the study, all of the men reported to a gymnastic hall, where they ate the same breakfast, weighed in, gave blood samples, and performed other tests such as grip-strength measurement. Then they had a simulated judo competition. The results were quite remarkable, though not surprising. Among those athletes who'd been on a restricted diet, blood chemistries were significantly altered (e.g., declines in testosterone and insulin; increases in cortisol and other compounds). Their physical performance was significantly affected, too, with poor results on tests of grip strength and horizontal rowing. This group also showed a decline in "vigor" and increases in fatigue and tension.

The authors of the study concluded that restricted nutrition "affects the physiology and psychology of judo athletes and impairs physical performance." Though I doubt we'll see a similar study of people who are ill or injured, the foregone conclusion is that diet would have a major impact on their ability to heal. In fact, it's reasonable to hypothesize that nutrition would have a far greater impact on this population than on supremely conditioned athletes.

The Pros and Cons of Taking Supplements

Taking nutritional supplements that contain megadoses of vitamins, minerals, and other nutrients is controversial. Generally, I don't recommend it. There are exceptions, however. So if you are taking supplements now or thinking of starting a regimen, talk with your doctor about what is best for you.

The easiest and best way to ensure that your body gets the many nutrients that it needs to heal optimally is to eat a varied and nutritious diet. Taking a lot of supplements may not be a good idea for a number of reasons. For example, you may be using a dose that is excessive (adhering to the principle of "if a little is good, then more is better"). The supplement may contain other ingredients that are harmful for you, or it may be missing ingredients that are necessary for another substance to do its job. Another possibility is that the supplement will interact with a prescription medication, rendering it less effective. (St. John's wort is among a number of supplements that interact with many prescription drugs.)

I have always been fascinated by the concept of "if a little is good, then more is better." While this may hold true for money, it definitely doesn't apply for what you put in your body. Nevertheless, many people—either knowingly or unwittingly—take megadoses of supplements, erroneously believing that it's good for them.

One of my patients is a Catholic nun who took a vow of poverty. What little money she has she spends on supplements. One day she brought in a shopping bag full of what she takes on a daily basis. After examining the various pills, I showed her that she was well above 100 percent of the Recommended Daily Allowances (RDAs). In fact, for several vitamins, she was taking as much as 5,000 percent of the RDAs. Multiply that by 365 days a year, and she was just under two million times the RDAs.

It's hard to imagine a scenario in which someone would need nearly two million extra doses of a vitamin in a given year. Moreover—and this is borne out by research studies—it's quite likely that megadosing can have some serious adverse health effects.

When I pointed all this out to my patient, she instantly realized that she was taking huge amounts of unnecessary and potentially harmful supplements. She assured me that she wouldn't buy any more—but being the frugal woman that she is, she would finish her current supply so that the money she had spent on them "wouldn't go to waste."

I do want to point out that supplements are not the only way in which megadosing can occur. For example, foods and beverages that are fortified with vitamins and minerals may pose a problem if the doses are too high. Some of these products are marketed as "functional foods" that are healthier choices because they are fortified. Again, though, too much of a good thing is not always such a good thing.

Megadosing isn't the only concern about supplements. Even if you take a reasonable amount of a given product, there still is the potential for serious side effects. One study conducted by Robert Saper, MD, and his colleagues at Harvard Medical School found significant and potentially quite toxic levels of heavy metals in certain Ayurvedic herbal medicine products. The results of this study, which appeared in the highly respected *Journal of the American Medical Association,* are as follows:

> Lead, mercury, and arsenic intoxication have been associated with the use of Ayurvedic herbal medicine products. . . . One of 5 Ayurvedic herbal medicine products produced in South Asia and available in Boston South Asian grocery stores contains potentially harmful levels of lead, mercury, and/or arsenic. Users of Ayurvedic medicine may be at risk for heavy metal toxicity, and testing of Ayurvedic herbal medicine products for toxic heavy metals should be mandatory.

Supplements—whether in the form of vitamins and minerals, herbs, Ayurvedic products, or other substances—are not subject to federal regulation and may contain ingredients that are not healthy. Some people think that because they purchase a product in a health food store, the product is safe and is good for them. This is not true. It's important to use all supplements cautiously. This goes back to my main point, which is that the best way to ensure that your body gets the nutrients it needs to heal optimally is to eat a varied and nutritious diet.

The one supplement that I routinely recommend is a single multivitamin, as an "insurance policy" that you're getting all of the essential vitamins and minerals in your diet. Look for a product that supplies 100 percent of the RDAs (it will say so on the label). Avoid those that have much higher amounts or that promote antioxidants or other substances. (We'll talk more about multivitamins a bit later in the chapter.)

I definitely am not opposed to using supplements. It is the misuse and overuse that I caution against. There are many supplements that doctors will recommend based on scientific literature that supports their use. For example, one study involving a combination of fish oil (omega-3 fatty acids) and olive oil showed significant improvement in joint pain, morning stiffness, and grip strength in people with rheumatoid arthritis. According to another study, fish oil may confer some benefit in patients with multiple sclerosis. I recommend supplements in very specific cases (e.g., additional calcium and vitamin D for patients at risk for osteoporosis, iron for someone who is anemic from an iron deficiency). But before you take any supplements, I urge you to talk with your doctor about whether they are necessary and what their potential benefits and risks may be.

8 Steps to a Super Healing Diet

There is no single perfect diet that we know of at this time. It's hard to imagine that there will ever be one that's appropriate for a population that encompasses so many different ethnic backgrounds, geographic origins, and individual food preferences. Instead, the best diet likely will always be one that involves eating a variety of nutritious foods.

Of course, this advice is too general to be very helpful. So in this section, I will offer more specific tips that will guide you in creating your personal Super Healing Diet. No matter what you like to eat, you can use food to help you physically recover if you adhere to these eight simple rules.

1. Eat three small- to medium-size meals each day, along with two healthy snacks.

2. Be sure to get enough lean protein and complex carbohydrates in your diet.

3. Eat five or more servings of colorful fruits and vegetables daily.

4. Talk with your doctor and a registered dietitian if you need to gain or lose weight.

5. Take a daily multivitamin, and get enough calcium and vitamin D.

6. Drink plenty of water.

7. Try to eat certified organic foods whenever possible.

8. Avoid nicotine completely and alcohol as much as possible.

When you determine your short- and long-term dietary goals (see opposite page), focus on those areas in which you feel you need to make the most improvement.

Step 1: Eat three small- to medium-size meals each day, along with two healthy snacks.

After a serious illness or injury, one of the most common complaints is profound fatigue. This can be the result of many factors, which I'll explain in more detail in the next chapter. One important consideration in treating fatigue is the role of food in energy.

Short- and Long-Term Dietary Goals

Though there is no perfect diet, there are some nutritional strategies that will help you heal optimally. You can construct your goals to reflect these strategies. The following lists might give you some ideas for goals—though they're meant only as reference points for your own Super Healing Plan.

Short-Term

- Eat three meals a day, plus two nutritious snacks.
- Switch all white bread to whole wheat bread.
- Eat at least three servings of fruits and vegetables daily.
- Make an appointment with your doctor or registered dietitian for nutrition advice.
- Take a multivitamin daily.
- Drink six glasses of water daily.
- Begin to read labels and purchase organic foods whenever possible.
- Reduce alcohol consumption to no more than three drinks weekly.

Long-Term

- Continue to eat three meals a day, plus two nutritious snacks.
- Switch from simple carbohydrates to complex carbs almost exclusively.
- Eat at least five, and ideally nine, servings of fruits and vegetables daily.
- Follow up with your doctor or dietitian at least once or twice, focusing specifically on nutrition advice.
- Take a multivitamin daily, and find out whether you should be taking calcium and vitamin D supplements and in what dosages.
- Continue to drink at least six glasses of water a day.
- Continue to replace conventional foods with organic foods whenever possible.
- Stop smoking.

Food, of course, is your body's fuel. Keeping your tank full without overindulging is important. Compare it to driving your car. How often do you let your gas tank go to empty so you run out of fuel in the middle of your ride? If you are like most people, you very rarely if ever do that. Instead, you keep at least a little gas in your tank at all times so you never run out.

It works well to do the same for your body. You don't want to eat so much at once that it causes a big spike in blood sugar followed a short time later by a big drop, which has a bottoming out effect on your energy level. Instead, if you eat to fuel your body so that you have a consistent and stable energy level, you'll feel better and you'll heal better. (If you have a medical condition with special dietary concerns, including diabetes, you should check with your doctor before making any dietary changes.)

Step 2: Be sure to get enough protein and complex carbohydrates.

Both protein and carbohydrates are good energy sources for your body. Carbohydrates are more readily available for conversion to energy, so it's important not to eliminate them from your diet. In fact, according to current dietary recommendations, between 45 and 65 percent of your calories should come from carbohydrate sources. (Fifteen to 20 percent should come from protein and 20 to 35 percent from fat—primarily "good fats" such as monounsaturates and polyunsaturates.)

Generally, carbohydrates fall into two categories: complex carbs, which include vegetables, beans and legumes, and whole grains; and simple carbs, such as breads, pastas, and other starches. Sometimes you might hear mention of a third category that contains sugars (e.g., table sugar, honey, and sweets such as candy).

All carbohydrates are broken down into sugar during the digestive process. As this sugar enters the bloodstream, the pancreas responds by releasing insulin to lower the blood sugar level. Scientists have devised a way to measure how fast and how high a particular food can make blood sugar rise. This is known as a food's glycemic index. You want to eat foods that have a low glycemic index because they don't cause such rapid and steep fluctuations in blood sugar levels. Complex carbohydrates fit this description.

You'll find a list of complex carbohydrate sources on the opposite page. Among them are whole grains, which differ from refined grains in that they retain the germ (the sprout of a new plant), endosperm (the energy source for the seed), and bran (the outer layer). To make refined grains such as white flour, the germ and bran—which contain important nutrients—are removed during the milling process. Some of the nutrients that may be lost

Complex Carbohydrate Sources

Complex carbohydrates are a good energy source, helping you to heal and feel less fatigued. As with the rest of your diet, try to get complex carbs from a variety of foods. Listed here are some examples.

- Arborio rice
- Barley
- Basmati rice
- Black, fava, kidney, lima, mung, navy, pinto, and white beans (these are high in protein, too)
- Bran
- Brown and wild rice
- Bulgur
- Chickpeas
- Flaxseed
- Fruits
- Kasha
- Millet
- Oats
- Rye
- Vegetables
- Whole grain breakfast cereal (100 percent)
- Whole grain wheat breads

include the B vitamins, vitamin E, iron, zinc, phytochemicals, and fiber. (Phytochemicals are rich in antioxidants and other healing substances. Examples include the anthocyanins in red, blue, and purple berries and the flavonones in citrus fruits and juices.)

Moreover, milling the grain means that it is digested more quickly, causing a faster and higher rise in blood sugar. Your body responds by releasing a large amount of insulin from the pancreas, which in turn causes a precipitous drop in blood sugar. This is exactly what you don't want when you are trying to heal well. You want a consistent blood sugar level rather than large spikes followed by dramatic dips.

Like carbohydrates, protein is an energy source. It also helps cells recover and regenerate. In certain cases, such as after extensive burns or during chemotherapy, the body has an increased need for protein to help with cellular recovery.

As I mentioned earlier, the current recommendation is to get about 15 to 20 percent of your calories from lean protein sources. For my patients healing from a serious injury or illness, I usually advise aiming for the higher end of the range—and sometimes even beyond. Depending on your medical condition, it's a good idea to talk with your doctor and a registered dietitian about your specific protein needs. There are ways to measure someone's protein status, which can be very helpful in cases of extensive cellular injury.

In terms of protein sources, plant-based proteins such as beans and nuts have some advantages over animal proteins. They provide vitamins, minerals, phytochemicals, beneficial fats, and fiber (which you can get only from plant-based foods). Beginning on page 94, you'll find a list of vegetarian protein sources (I include dairy in this category).

Step 3: Eat five or more servings of colorful fruits and vegetables daily.

Fruits and vegetables are quite remarkable for their many healing components. These foods are rich in vitamins, minerals, and other substances (such as phytochemicals) that help promote recovery. Eating at least five servings of fruits and vegetables each day is one of the best things you can do for your body. Examples of a single serving would be:

- One medium fruit
- ½ cup raw, frozen, or canned fruit (in 100 percent juice)
- ¼ cup dried fruit
- ½ cup raw, cooked, frozen, or canned vegetables
- 1 cup raw leafy vegetables
- ¾ cup 100 percent juice (fruit or vegetable)
- ½ cup cooked, frozen, or canned legumes (beans and peas)

By eating a diet rich in fruits and vegetables, you will get plenty of nutrients that support the healing process. One example is vitamin C, which has long been touted for its health benefits—and deservedly so. Vitamin C is essential for wound healing. In fact, a deficiency can lead to delayed wound healing along with increased blood vessel (capillary) fragility and a reduced ability to ward off infection. That said, megadoses of vitamin C—such as the 18,000 milligrams a day proposed by Linus Pauling—are not believed to be helpful and could prove harmful. While vitamin C deficiency slows healing, excessive doses (more than 2,000 milligrams per day) have not been shown to accelerate healing. This is why it's best to get your vitamin C from foods, not supplements.

Like vitamin C, zinc plays a role in wound healing. It also supports protein synthesis and immune function. Running low on zinc can lead to not only delayed wound healing and poor immune function but also loss of appetite. Again, if you eat plenty of fruits and vegetables, it is unlikely that you will experience a zinc deficiency. Taking too much zinc (in supplement form) can impede healing and may contribute to a copper deficiency, which can further undermine the healing process.

Fruits and vegetables also are good sources of antioxidants and phyto-chemicals. Diets rich in antioxidants appear to improve healing. Antioxidants such as vitamins C and E, beta-carotene, and lycopene are found in abundance in this food category. Lycopene—in tomatoes, apricots, guava, water-melon, papaya, and pink grapefruit—seems to be a particularly powerful antioxidant. As a general rule, darkly colored fruits and vegetables contain the most antioxidants and phytochemicals.

Other substances in fruits and vegetables promote healing as well. Among those that have been identified are carotenoids (in orange-colored foods such as carrots, yams, apricots, and cantaloupe), anthocyanins (in tomatoes, red peppers, and red grapefruit juice), and sulfides (in garlic and onions). Still others have yet to be discovered.

In some studies, fruit and vegetable supplements that come in pill form have been shown to raise antioxidant levels in the blood. The primary concern with these supplements is that while fruits and vegetables are known to help prevent certain kinds of cancer, scientists aren't exactly sure which constituents of these foods are most beneficial. Moreover, as mentioned above, fruits and vegetables likely contain more therapeutic substances than we currently know about. What this means is that fruit and vegetable supplements, while perhaps helpful, almost certainly are not as good as the actual foods. I generally recommend a supplement for my patients only when it is clear that they are not eating fruits and vegetables and are unable to change their diets to include more.

Step 4: Talk to your doctor and a registered dietitian if you need to gain or lose weight.

A patient of mine, Charlie Woodward, had been diagnosed with Merkel cell carcinoma and subsequently developed swelling in the affected leg (lymphedema). When I first saw him, he was having a lot of trouble getting around, in part because he needed to lose weight. His case was complicated by the fact that he needed to lose weight overall, but particularly in the fluid-filled leg. This meant that he had both fluid and extra adipose (fat) tissue to get rid of.

Vegetarian Protein Sources

To Super Heal, your body needs plenty of protein. It's best to choose lean sources and vary your choices as much as possible. Generally speaking, plant-based proteins are lean and nutritious. Nuts are fairly high in calories and fat, but it's mostly good fats (the monounsaturated and polyunsaturated types).

If you're limiting your consumption of meat and other animal-based proteins, you need to pay special attention to your intake of iron and vitamin B_{12}. Both are important for healing, but they can run low in a largely vegetarian diet. Some vegetarians eat animal products such as eggs and cheese, which are good protein sources but a bit higher in bad fats (saturates).

Vegetarian Sources of Protein

- Brown rice
- Cheeses
- Cottage cheese
- Eggs
- Legumes
- Lentils
- Meat analogs (e.g., veggie burgers)
- Nut and seed butters
- Nuts
- Quinoa
- Quorn products
- Seeds
- Soy milk
- Tempeh
- Tofu
- Yogurt

I referred Charlie to an excellent registered dietitian, who gave him dietary advice specific to his situation (e.g., reduce salt intake, take a daily multivitamin, and consume an appropriate number of calories). At the same time, Charlie met with a physical therapist who was able to help reduce the amount of fluid in his leg. Ultimately, Charlie lost more than 20 pounds, which made a real difference in his ability to move about as well as in his stamina and general well-being. You'll read Charlie's Remarkable Recovery story at the end of this chapter.

When you've been seriously ill or injured, it's smart to get professional advice about gaining or losing weight. In general, as with any diet, you

Vegetarian Sources of Iron

- Almonds
- Beans
- Bean sprouts
- Blackstrap molasses
- Bran
- Dried fruit
- Fortified cereals
- Leafy green vegetables
- Lentils
- Parsley
- Prune juice
- Sesame seeds
- Soybean nuts
- Spinach
- Whole grains
- Yeast extract

Vegetarian Sources of Vitamin B$_{12}$

- Alfalfa sprouts
- Blue-green algae (spirulina, chlorella) and seaweed
- Dairy
- Eggs
- Fortified soy milk
- Milk
- Miso
- Tamari
- Tempeh
- Yeast extract
- Yogurt

need to consider total number of calories as well as total grams of fat. Fat, along with protein and carbohydrates, is an energy source that your body needs to function well. Most people don't need to worry about getting more calories or fat. Actually, the trend has been to get too many calories and too much fat. For this reason, my usual advice is to stick with a low-fat diet, which also helps to control calorie intake, while in the Healing Zone.

There are instances in which someone has lost a lot of weight and is in need of replenishing fat stores. This person may need to increase both calorie intake and dietary fat content. Again, it's important to do this in consultation with a physician and/or registered dietitian.

In general, people should eat about 10 to 15 calories for each pound of body weight to maintain their current weight. If you're trying to gain, you'll need to eat additional calories. About 500 extra per day is a reasonable number to shoot for; this will add about 1 pound per week. If your goal is to lose, you'll need to trim your calorie intake. However, you should be sure to consume enough calories to keep up your energy level. If you don't, you may lose weight more quickly, but you'll feel lousy. You should lose weight gradually, so your energy level remains stable.

As for dietary fat, it's best to stick with small amounts of monounsaturated and polyunsaturated fats, the so-called "good fats." This group includes vegetable oils such as grape seed, corn, olive, and canola; nuts; and certain fish (e.g., salmon, lake trout, tuna, and herring). Saturated fats (in whole milk, cream, butter, and fatty meats) and trans fats (in margarine; vegetable shortening; and packaged breads, cakes, cookies, and crackers) are "bad fats." It's a good idea to limit consumption of these fats, if not avoid them altogether.

Step 5: Take a daily multivitamin, and get enough calcium and vitamin D.

Though not everyone needs a multivitamin, most people can benefit from taking one. As I mentioned earlier, choose a product that does not exceed 100 percent of the RDAs for the essential vitamins and minerals. There is no difference between natural and synthetic brands.

For those who are anemic because of an iron deficiency, a multivitamin can be especially helpful. But iron can contribute to constipation. If you don't have an iron deficiency, consider choosing a low-iron multivitamin (often labeled as a "senior" or geriatric alternative).

Also, pay attention to your calcium and vitamin D intake, especially if you have sustained a bone injury, such as a bruise or fracture. Both calcium and vitamin D support bone health. But individual needs for these nutrients can vary quite a bit based on gender, age, medical conditions, and other factors. If you have concerns about your bones, ask your doctor whether taking supplemental calcium and vitamin D would be helpful. Keep in mind, too, that weight-bearing exercise such as walking promotes stronger bones (unless you have a bone fracture that limits you to non- or partial-weight-bearing activity) and that caffeine, alcohol, and tobacco all have a negative impact on bone healing and bone density.

Step 6: Drink plenty of water.

Adequate hydration is critical to the healing process. Water and other fluids help keep blood circulating throughout your body, transporting important healing substances to your cells and organs while carrying away waste. Dehydration can result in poor wound healing and other uncomfortable side effects, including constipation.

For proper hydration, nothing beats water. Most people should drink six to eight 8-ounce glasses of water each day while they are in the Healing Zone. But do ask your doctor how much water you should be drinking; if you have kidney problems or congestive heart failure, that amount might be too much. On the other hand, it might be too little if you are on a very high-protein diet, have draining wounds, are vomiting a lot, or have a chronic fever.

Step 7: Try to eat certified organic foods whenever possible.

We don't know very much about the long-term effects of the chemicals used to help grow or preserve food. In the future, we will find out whether things such as bovine growth hormone, irradiation, and genetically engineered

Eating to Improve Energy

What you eat can affect your energy level. In order to heal optimally, you'll want to have as much energy as possible. If you've been battling fatigue, try incorporating these tips into your Super Healing Plan.

- Make sure to get enough complex carbohydrates and protein in your diet.
- Don't skip any meals.
- Try eating three small to medium meals each day, with two nutritious snacks in between.
- Avoid refined sugar and simple carbohydrates (such as sweets, crackers, and chips). These can provide a quick energy boost by spiking your blood sugar, but it's followed by a precipitous drop that can leave you feeling tired and sluggish.
- Get enough calories.
- If you are anemic, try to eat more iron-rich foods.
- Stay well hydrated. The best drinks for hydration are water, fruit and vegetable juices, and milk. It is best to avoid or limit consumption of caffeinated drinks (including coffees and teas), sodas, and alcohol.

food either are not particularly harmful or can contribute to serious health problems. It seems unlikely that these things will turn out to be good for us. Therefore, when people ask me whether they should eat organic or conventional food, my answer is that they would be wise to incorporate as much certified organic food into their diets as possible.

Certified organic food, though sometimes more expensive than conventional food, is grown with a number of restrictions. For example, organic farmers in the meat industry don't feed antibiotics or growth hormones to their animals. Organic food also is devoid of conventional pesticides, fertilizers, and ionizing radiation. Some studies have shown that organic crops may be higher in phytochemicals than conventionally grown crops.

The National Organic Program (NOP) is a federal law that requires all organic food products to meet the same standards and be certified via the same process. Only products labeled as organic have met USDA organic standards. ("Natural" is not the same as "organic.") Along with the NOP, the USDA has developed strict labeling rules to inform consumers about the specific content of the organic food they buy. The USDA Organic seal means that at least 95 percent of a product is organic.

Keep in mind, though, that it's better to eat conventional food—especially fruits and vegetables—than to skip them altogether because they're not certified as organic. If organic produce is not an option because of availability or cost, be sure to wash fruits and vegetables thoroughly under clean, cold, running water before eating them—even if you're planning to peel, cut, or cook them. Use a scrub brush when appropriate and discard any outer leaves when possible, as they tend to be higher in pesticide residues. Steer clear of rinses, soaps, and chlorine bleach solutions.

Step 8: Avoid nicotine completely and alcohol as much as possible.

Nicotine, especially in the form of cigarettes, is very toxic to healing tissues. Many studies have shown that smoking prevents optimal recovery. In a review article titled "Cutaneous Effects of Smoking" that appeared in the *Journal of Cutaneous Medicine and Surgery,* the authors explain: "Smoking has been shown to significantly decrease the immune response, leading to poor wound healing. In particular, smoking decreases interleukin-1 production, inhibits the early signals for B-cell transduction pathways, decreases cytotoxicity of natural killer cells, and causes T-cell anergy."

What all this means is that smoking undermines immune function in a number of ways that can disrupt the healing process. Further, nicotine is a toxin that not only directly affects the immune system but also indirectly slows or prevents healing by reducing blood flow to the injured area.

Most people begin smoking in their youth, when they are most vulnerable, least knowledgeable, and years away from realizing any of the ill effects of nicotine. When I talk with my patients about smoking, I always tread lightly. I know that they beat themselves up over this issue, and the last thing I want to do is to cause them more distress.

If you smoke and you want to quit, rather than focusing on past attempts that have not resulted in lasting abstinence, keep in mind that the road to success typically includes stretches in which someone has stopped smoking—whether for a day, a month, or a year. This also applies to those quitting chewing tobacco and snuff. Therefore, if you have been able to stop smoking in the past, even for a short period, you have had some success. Moreover, this probably is a time in your life when you are extremely motivated to kick the tobacco habit. That, along with your past short-term successes, can be the key to stopping smoking for good.

Alcohol is a misunderstood and misrepresented substance that definitely is not helpful in healing from serious injury or illness. Though some studies suggest that alcohol in unknown but probably quite small quantities may be somewhat helpful in preventing heart disease, a much larger body of research recognizes alcohol's very harmful effects. In particular, alcohol has been linked to a number of serious medical conditions, including dementia, liver cirrhosis, and cancer. Since this is a book about physical healing, I will focus on how alcohol hinders this process.

One of the effects of alcohol is that it is toxic to nerves. Therefore, if you have an illness or injury that has compromised your nerve function, it's important not to add a nerve toxin to your body. In all likelihood, your nerves will heal better and more completely if you don't imbibe.

Alcohol also undermines immune function, in part because of its impact on cytokines. These chemicals, which are produced by our bodies, help to regulate both the immune system and the healing process. In a research article titled "Cytokines and Alcohol," the authors noted, "Alcohol use alters immune defenses against infections and results in increased incidence of bacterial pneumonias, a higher rate of chronic hepatitis C infections, and increased susceptibility to HIV infection." While these particular medical conditions may not be of concern to you, it's important to recognize that alcohol travels throughout your body and may worsen damage to already injured cells and organs.

Sometimes people turn to alcohol for "medicinal reasons"—for example, to help control their mood, reduce stress, or relieve pain. Alcohol is not good medicine; in fact, it may have the opposite effect (e.g., instead of improving mood, it can work as a depressant and leave a person feeling even worse). If you are using alcohol in a medicinal manner, talk with your doctor about alternative strategies that would be more helpful.

Eating to Improve Mood

What you eat can influence how you feel emotionally. The better you feel, the easier time you will have working your Super Healing Plan. Consider these dietary strategies to boost your mood.

- Eat regularly and don't skip meals.
- Avoid alcohol.
- Limit caffeine.
- Steer clear of refined sugar and simple carbohydrates such as sweets, crackers, and chips. These may give you a bit of an emotional lift, but as your blood sugar dips, so can your mood.

Though I don't advocate drinking alcohol if you are in the Healing Zone, it is unlikely that an occasional alcoholic beverage or two will do any harm. Alcohol seems to be the most detrimental in those who drink occasionally in excess as well as those who drink regularly, even in moderation. Therefore, if you drink in moderation on special occasions only, it likely will not affect your ability to heal well.

Use Your Diet to Super Heal

I often give motivational speeches on healing. I enjoy the challenge of imparting an important message while at the same time choosing language and stories to entertain. One event I went to was in a big theater in Ohio. My appearance was part of a lecture series that had been going on for more than 50 years. The event coordinators told me, "Most of the people we invite to speak are really famous. You're not. So you'll have to make sure that you offer the audience really meaningful information."

I had just 40 minutes for my presentation, which would be about how to heal optimally. Since diet is one of the three most important factors in healing, I shared some of the same information that appears in this chapter. The event was followed by a luncheon. One woman with pure white hair, sparkling eyes, and a bounce in her step came up to me and commented, "Dearie, I liked what you said, but I'm 86 years old and healthy. I'm going to keep taking all of my supplements, and I'm not going to follow any of your advice."

Rather than being offended, I actually enjoy when people come up to me and (usually very politely) tell me things like that. The truth is that whether it's genes or diet or supplements or whatever, this woman is doing well and doesn't need to follow my advice. But, as I gently explained to this lovely lady, my recommendations are not for healthy 86-year-old women. They're for those who are in need of healing.

If you are working toward better health, certainly consider the information in this chapter. More important, pay attention to what you are putting into your body and how it affects your ability to heal optimally.

REMARKABLE RECOVERY

Charles Woodward

I was diagnosed with Merkel cell carcinoma, a form of skin cancer that probably was caused by sun exposure to my leg. I had to have surgical excisions, which got rid of most of the cancer. But in the meantime we found out that it had spread to the lymph nodes in my groin area. I believe it came out to be a stage 3 cancer, so it was very, very difficult to get through that situation.

I've got two boys who are grown—one's married—and my wife. I've been absolutely healthy all my life. I don't even remember having the flu. I was a paratrooper in the service, and I've always been very physically fit and able to do anything. When this came about, it was unbelievable to realize that at 57 years old, a sunburn sometime in my life caused this little lump on my leg, and it was going to take my life, and my whole future was gone. One doctor said I might live 2 years; another said I would have 6 months. This was very devastating to me. I immediately panicked, and I was so overwhelmed with sadness that I just didn't know what to do.

My son went online and found out the seriousness of Merkel cell—that it spreads like wildfire. I had begun getting all my affairs in order. Then I found an oncologist who was very experienced with this type of cancer, and he said, "Look, this is what we're going to do. I want to treat you just as if you were my family member. You're young enough, you're strong enough, to withstand a lot of the chemo and the battle with the radiation that you're going to have to endure." He said, "It may be real hard to do, but this is what's going to work." And I did it.

I've been cancer free for several years now, but I developed a problem with swelling in my leg, called lymphedema. It got really bad, and I was waiting for my leg to explode or for the blood circulation to cut off. I was saying to myself, "Okay, this is what's going to happen, and I have to live with it and possibly lose a leg." At my first appointment with Dr. Silver, she told me that her team could help, and I wouldn't lose my leg.

I went through the oncology rehab program, and they told me how to exercise. I've lost more than 20 pounds. The physical thera- pist I worked with said, "This is what we're going to do," and she gave me a plan. I saw her for 2 months. I had to drive a long way, but I could have cared less about the time and the gas. I said, "I am getting results." I couldn't believe how nice I felt. I wouldn't have changed anything.

When I went to see my oncologist, he was absolutely blown away, because he had seen the before and this was after. He was just abso- lutely astonished. He couldn't believe the success. I still have to wrap

Serotonin and Diet

Serotonin, a naturally occurring chemical in our bodies, has a signifi- cant effect on mood and appetite. Most of the antidepressant medica- tions prescribed today work by raising serotonin levels in the brain.

There are many reasons that serotonin may be a bit low in someone who is in the Healing Zone. In studies, researchers have explored how tryptophan and tyrosine—both large-chain amino acids that are precursors to serotonin—affect mood. For example, the drug inter- feron is known to cause depression in some people. Interferon is used to treat a variety of conditions, including hepatitis C and multiple myeloma. Studies have revealed that people who take this drug tend to show reductions in their tryptophan levels.

Researchers also are investigating how diets either rich or poor in these amino acids affect mood. In one study, participants who ingested 1 gram of tryptophan were significantly less "quarrelsome" than those who took a placebo. Other studies have suggested that tryptophan and tyrosine can improve depression in those susceptible to it.

Diet is not the only way to treat mood problems; some people may be better off using prescription antidepressants, for example. But clearly, there are significant links between what we put in our bodies and how we feel emotionally. A diet that's very rich in tryptophan and tyrosine also tends to be high in carbohydrates and low in protein, my leg every night and put a pressure stocking on during the day, but it's just been a wonderful, wonderful situation. It was the best thing I ever did—getting rehabilitation.

Because of my family, I'm just too young to see the other side right now. So far everything has worked and worked and worked, and it's an absolute success in my case. When I was diagnosed with cancer, I looked at the faces of my grandkids and my sons and my wife, and I said, "Vietnam didn't get me, and I'm going to fight this to the end." That's what I ended up doing—giving it the whole shot. And it worked. You just can't give up; you've got to fight with everything you have. I've had a remarkable recovery.

which isn't necessarily ideal for people going through the Healing Zone.

Below are foods that may help raise serotonin levels in your brain. However, if you are depressed, anxious, or very stressed, make a point of talking with your doctor about how you're feeling.

High Serotonin Concentration

- Banana
- Kiwi
- Pineapple
- Plantain
- Plums
- Tomatoes

Moderate Serotonin Concentration

- Avocados
- Black olives
- Broccoli
- Cantaloupe
- Cauliflower
- Dates
- Eggplant
- Figs
- Grapefruit
- Honeydew melon
- Spinach

Chapter 7

Rest to Recover

In order to heal optimally, you need to sleep well. Sleep is so important, in fact, that it is the third key component of your Super Healing Plan. Without proper rest, your body cannot adequately recover from illness or injury. But while it's easy to say that both the quality and quantity of your sleep matter, it's not so easy to ensure that you are getting what you need.

Poor sleep is practically synonymous with serious illness. Where one exists, so does the other. Nevertheless, you can do a lot to facilitate the healing process by focusing on ways to get proper sleep. In this chapter, I'll explain how to improve your ability to rest so your body can mend.

It's long been known that good health depends on proper sleep. Recently, though, sleep has become such a significant public health issue that if you aren't getting enough, you could quite literally be prosecuted and sent to prison for it.

If you think I'm exaggerating, let me tell you a story about a woman I once worked with. I'll call her Joyce. The two of us were attending a medical conference that had begun early in the morning and lasted until late in the afternoon. Afterward, I drove home alone. On my way, I passed a terrible accident that had occurred on the opposite side of the interstate, backing up traffic for miles. I didn't think much of it until later, when I heard that Joyce—traveling the same route home as I—had somehow crossed over the center barrier and collided head-on with a van carrying a father and two children. Joyce sustained bone fractures and skin lacerations. I don't know what happened to the others, though apparently all of them were injured. Joyce, who was sober at the time of the accident, was charged with reckless driving. Part of the prosecution's case centered on the belief that Joyce had been driving while overly tired.

Fatigue can be a criminal offense under the right circumstances—

usually when a vehicular or industrial accident occurs and it's suspected that the person responsible was too tired to perform optimally. Major industrial catastrophes such as Chernobyl and Three Mile Island, as well as serious accidents such as the *Exxon Valdez* and the space shuttle *Challenger,* have been attributed in part to sleepiness in the workplace. When it comes to "drowsy drivers," the article "Fatigue and the Criminal Law" notes that though most countries and states don't have laws regulating fatigue, tired drivers who get into accidents can be prosecuted under various other statutes, such as reckless or dangerous driving.

New Jersey, recognizing that excessive sleepiness is the second leading cause of car accidents and a major cause of truck accidents in the United States, has been more aggressive about addressing this problem than most states. It's a criminal offense for a person who has not slept in the previous 24 hours to drive. The law can be invoked if the driver is involved in a motor vehicle accident and the crash results in a death.

Studies have shown that sleepy drivers are just as dangerous as drunk drivers. According to an article titled "Sleep Deprivation," which appeared in the medical journal *Primary Care: Clinics in Office Practice,* "Subjects who drove after being awake for 17 to 19 hours performed worse than those who had a blood alcohol level of 0.05 percent. Twenty to 25 hours of wakefulness produces performance decrements equivalent to those observed at a blood alcohol concentration of 0.10 percent, a level deemed unsafe and unacceptable when working or driving."

Sleep is so incredibly important for physical and mental restoration that without proper rest, we don't function well. Optimal physical healing, regardless of the underlying illness or injury, requires excellent sleep. Our bodies know this intuitively. Consider the two things that happen without fail when you have an acute infection: You get a fever, and you sleep more. These are the body's natural defenses against infection.

But sleeping well does much more than fight infection. It helps you to physically heal as a variety of concerted chemical reactions take place while you're least aware that they're happening. Among its myriad benefits, sleep:

- Slows metabolism and conserves energy
- Cools the body and the brain
- Improves immune function
- Replenishes glycogen and other energy stores
- Promotes and reorganizes memory
- Allows for rehearsal of new learning
- Enables emotional adjustment through dreams

Why Good Sleep Helps You Heal

Sleep is a complicated process; much remains to be learned about what happens during the time that we are at rest. All mammals sleep, though in radically different amounts and in various ways. For example, in order to avoid drowning, aquatic mammals sleep on one side of their brain at a time.

Ideally, humans should get a solid 7 to 8 hours of sleep each night. Your sleep is divided into two main stages: non–rapid eye movement (non-REM) and rapid eye movement (REM). Non-REM is quiet sleep, while REM is more active. This is when you dream.

Approximately 75 percent of your night should be spent in non-REM sleep. It occurs first and is believed to have the greatest impact on immune function and healing. Non-REM sleep is further divided into four stages, beginning with stage 1, when you are just falling asleep and in between sleep and wakefulness. Then you advance through the other stages until you reach stage 4, in which brain waves show the highest level of slow-wave activity.

Slow-wave sleep is considered to be the most restorative, so you want to encourage slow-wave sleep in order to recover optimally. One theory behind why this type of sleep supports healing is that your body literally slows down, cools off, and lowers its metabolic demand—allowing your body to truly rest and replenish its energy stores. At the end of stage 4 of non-REM sleep, you transition to REM sleep. Then you repeat the entire cycle, which lasts about 90 minutes. You continue repeating the cycle throughout the night.

The body's overall sleep-awake cycle tends to operate in 24-hour increments. This is what's known as your *circadian rhythm*, or your biological clock.

While you're sleeping, your body functions differently than while you are awake. For example, your body makes a chemical called serotonin that can influence your mood. As I mentioned in the previous chapter, many of the popular prescription medications for depression are in a class known as selective serotonin reuptake inhibitors. In other words, they allow more serotonin to be present in the brain, thus improving mood. The activity of the serotoninergic system in your body changes depending on whether you are asleep or awake. Though there is much to sort out about how sleep affects serotonin levels and how this in turn affects depression, we know that there is a strong connection among the three.

Proper sleep also facilitates what is known as brain plasticity. In other words, it encourages your brain to be agile and facile and to work well, not only improving your memory and concentration but also helping the brain to heal after an injury.

In healthy people, sleep deprivation—commonly known as *sleep debt*, when your body needs more sleep than it is getting—alters metabolism during the waking hours and promotes premature aging. It also can lead to a state similar to diabetes. In fact, sleep has such a significant effect on blood sugar (glucose) metabolism that some studies suggest certain people may be at higher risk for diabetes if they aren't sleeping well. In those who've been diagnosed with diabetes, poor sleep may cause such a significant and persistent issue with blood sugar control that it can alter the progression of the disease.

What Happens to Sleep after an Injury or Illness

The vast majority of people who are in the midst of or recently experienced a serious illness or injury have sleep problems. Poor sleep is a component of the Triple Threat to optimal healing, while sleeping well fosters Super Healing Synergy. (For a refresher on these concepts, see page 23.)

The immune system, which is of paramount importance in healing, suffers in the presence of too little sleep, poor-quality sleep, or fragmented/interrupted sleep. In this regard, there is much we know and much we still have to learn. We know that wounds heal more slowly when sleep deprivation occurs. We also know that the brain is the primary organ affected by sleep and that it releases various chemicals and immune products that directly influence other parts of the body, including the immune system. In a report titled "Neuroimmunologic Aspects of Sleep and Sleep Loss," published in *Seminars in Clinical Neuropsychiatry*, researchers note, "The complex and intimate interactions between the sleep and immune systems have been the focus of study for several years. Immune factors, particularly the interleukins, regulate sleep and in turn are altered by sleep and sleep deprivation."

As I mentioned earlier, the sleep-brain relationship is extremely complex, and many chemical reactions occur simultaneously during the nighttime hours. One involves changes in secretion of the hormone melatonin, which is thought to enhance immune function and healing. The brain produces greater quantities of melatonin at night, during sleep. If you aren't getting proper rest, your melatonin supply may suffer.

You may be wondering whether a simple solution would be to take a melatonin supplement. It's not quite so simple. At this point, it is impossible to predict how much melatonin you would need and whether your body would use it in the same manner as the melatonin your brain naturally produces. Besides, melatonin is just one compound; many others may play a role. So while taking supplements may be appealing, the truly simple solution—and the most effective—is to sleep enough and sleep well.

Research shows that sleep problems often begin or worsen in the hospital environment, which can be a difficult place to rest and recuperate. A report titled "Sleep in the Intensive Care Unit," which appeared in the journal *Pharmacotherapy,* noted that the average amount of sleep for a patient in an ICU setting is less than 2 hours a day.

Hospitals are noisy places, with people and machines that contribute to continuous sleep interruptions. A report by the World Health Organization recommended that hospital noise levels be no higher than 35 decibels at night and no higher than 40 decibels during the day. But in one study of a general surgical ward, noise levels reached 70 decibels during the day. The lowest level was 36, which occurred during the midnight to 7:00 a.m. shift. This still is slightly higher than WHO's recommended maximum nighttime noise level of 35 decibels.

Hospitals are where many patients begin the healing process, and health professionals gradually are coming to understand how the hospital environment might undermine healing by interfering with good-quality sleep. However, according to anesthesiologist William Peruzzi, MD, who wrote the report about sleep in the ICU, "The importance of sleep for patients who are critically ill is frequently overlooked by even the most astute clinicians."

How Poor Sleep Disrupts Healing

Constant interruptions and noisy wards are not the only reasons that hospital patients get such poor sleep. Emotional distress certainly can contribute to difficulty falling asleep or staying asleep, as can pain from injuries or surgical incisions. Hot flashes and the urge to urinate can cause frequent awakenings. Poor sleep is a common side effect of certain medications. The combination of lack of exercise, lying in bed most of the day, and taking naps can disrupt the body's normal sleep-wake cycle.

These same factors can come into play for people who are healing from illness or injury outside the hospital setting. No matter where or why it begins, insomnia—difficulty falling asleep or staying asleep—contributes to suboptimal physical recovery.

Sometimes poor sleep can result from an underlying medical condition such as sleep apnea, in which breathing halts for short periods during the sleep cycle. Often the person has no idea that it's happening.

One of my patients is a woman in her forties who was diagnosed with breast cancer several years ago. More than a year before her diagnosis, she complained of profound fatigue—a symptom she later attributed to her as-yet-undetected malignancy. She underwent surgery, followed by chemo-therapy and radiation. Not surprisingly, her fatigue became worse.

When I first met with this patient 4 years after her diagnosis, her primary symptom was debilitating fatigue that permeated every aspect of her life, including her work. Before coming to me, she had sought out several medical opinions, virtually all of which pointed to chronic fatigue syndrome as the source of her problem.

During the course of her workup, this patient underwent a sleep study, which is an excellent objective measure of just what happens while someone is asleep. I highly recommend a sleep study for people with prolonged fatigue. In my patient's case, her study showed that she had "mild" sleep apnea, a condition characterized by pauses in breathing. Both my patient and her previous doctors discounted this finding as insignificant. But in my mind, there was a reasonable chance that this woman's profound fatigue—which had begun before her cancer diagnosis—was caused by her sleep apnea. Her cancer treatment only compounded a preexisting problem.

This patient was truly suffering, and her lack of energy was having a very negative effect on her quality of life. "Why not treat your sleep apnea and see how much better you feel?" I asked her. She immediately agreed. As I suspected, she responded well to treatment, which for her included wearing a nighttime face mask connected to a breathing machine. While she still felt tired at times, her energy improved markedly.

Proper rest is essential in all cases of serious illness. For those undergoing heart surgery, however, it takes on even greater importance. In fact, it could save lives. Approximately 7 of every 10 patients who undergo heart bypass surgery complain of sleep problems in the first few weeks after discharge. For many of these patients, poor sleep continues for months. This has serious implications for cardiac patients because it can lead to rises in heart rate and blood pressure, both of which cause unnecessary strain on the heart and may put it at risk for further injury.

One of my patients, David Rubin, experienced this firsthand on September 11, 2006, when he was on board an airplane traveling from San Francisco to Boston. En route, his heart suddenly stopped. Fortunately, he was resuscitated, but he ended up needing open-heart surgery. In our first phone conversation after the operation, I told him that one of the most important things for him to focus on was getting enough good-quality sleep.

I have known David for many years; though he had just turned 80 at the time of his fateful flight, he was (and is) an active and highly successful businessman in the Boston community. He also is extremely busy, and I know that he rarely sleeps as much as he should. In fact, he says that prior to his heart surgery, he "never slept more than 6 hours a night." Several weeks after his operation, I asked how much he was sleeping. He said, "Since the heart surgery, I'm sleeping more like 7½ to 8 hours, which I think is helpful for my recovery. Generally, though, I don't like to slow down and rest." (David's Remarkable Recovery story appears at the end of this chapter.)

How Sleep Affects Chronic Medical Conditions

David's story is dramatic and traumatic—literally, a heart-stopping experience. While proper sleep can help people like David recover from sudden illness or injury, it is no less important for those who are living with chronic medical conditions.

Unfortunately, chronic conditions have a well-deserved reputation for wreaking havoc with sleep patterns. For example, in a study evaluating the sleep patterns of people with early-stage chronic kidney disease, researchers identified sleep disorders in more than 80 percent of the participants. The reasons for this are many, including altered levels of blood urea, creatinine, and parathyroid hormone, as well as the presence of anemia and difficulty regulating blood pressure.

Another study evaluated the extent of sleep problems in women with systemic lupus erythematosus (also known as lupus). More than 50 percent of the women reported moderate to severe sleep impairment. In a separate study assessing the impact of pain on sleep in people with chronic low back pain, researchers observed a 55 percent increase in reports of sleep problems after the onset of pain.

I treat many people with chronic conditions who are traveling through the Healing Zone. While there is no cure for their conditions at this time, rehabilitative interventions can be extraordinarily helpful. Ensuring the best possible rest is one of the interventions that can vastly improve quality of life, despite chronic illness.

One of my patients is a lovely gentleman who is a polio survivor. He has five grown children and many grandchildren, as well as a successful law practice that keeps him extremely active. When he came to see me a couple of years ago, he thought that he might be suffering from a severe case of post-polio syndrome, a chronic medical condition that occurs in some polio survivors many years after the initial viral infection. One of the hallmark symptoms is unusual and debilitating fatigue, and this gentleman complained of feeling incredibly tired during the day.

Sleep disorders such as sleep apnea are common in polio survivors who are experiencing fatigue. In a study conducted by my friend Daria Trojan, MD, and her colleagues, sleep-disordered breathing was present in 65 percent of polio survivors who reported fatigue as a symptom.

When my patient said that he was extremely tired, I did what I always do for people who complain of daytime fatigue that interferes with their ability to function: I ordered a sleep study. This patient's study revealed that he had severe sleep apnea. I referred him to a sleep specialist, who suggested that he try a breathing machine similar to the one used by my young breast cancer patient who responded so favorably to treatment. It's called CPAP, short for continuous positive airway pressure.

Within 6 months, this gentleman felt much, much better. Though he still was experiencing some minor symptoms of post-polio syndrome, his state of health and quality of life showed dramatic improvement with proper rest.

Short- and Long-Term Sleep Goals

Below are several examples of short-term goals that can advance you toward a long-term goal of regularly getting at least 8 hours of quality sleep each night and not feeling unusually tired during the day. Again, these are just ideas for your consideration. Create your own goals in a manner that will work best for you.

Short-Term

- Avoid caffeine after 3:00 p.m.
- Reduce wine consumption from one to two glasses in the evening to no more than one.
- Make an appointment to talk with your doctor about sleep and fatigue.
- Review your medications with your pharmacist and determine which ones may be affecting your sleep.
- Give up taking naps during the day.
- Plan for a 15- to 30-minute rest period daily.

Long-Term

Your long-term goal is to regularly get at least 8 hours of good-quality sleep. If you aren't able to achieve this by the first 6-month mark, then repeat it as your long-term goal for the second 6 months. Continue with your short-term goals in the meantime. You also might talk with your doctor about the possibility of a sleep study.

Many of my patients with chronic medical conditions, who follow their own versions of the Super Healing Plan, feel as though they've experienced a "miraculous" shift in their health status, despite the fact that they haven't been cured in the conventional sense. Sleep is incredibly important for optimal health and healing, no matter if the underlying illness is acute or chronic.

Steps to Take to Improve Sleep

To correct poor sleep, one of the first and most important steps is to simply recognize the problem. Some people know that they aren't getting enough sleep or the right kind of sleep. Others aren't so sure. During office visits with my patients, I routinely ask questions about sleep, napping, daytime fatigue, memory and concentration, and mood. The answers to questions on these topics can provide important clues about how well someone is resting.

One thing I've noticed is that people often are mistaken about how well they're sleeping at night. I've had literally hundreds of conversations with patients who come to their office visits with their sleep partners. When I ask the patient if he or she snores or tosses and turns at night, the patient usually says no. But out of the corner of my eye, I'll catch a surprised look on the face of the partner, who will contradict what the patient just said. This means that no matter what your impression of how you are sleeping, you can't possibly know if it's accurate.

You may be thinking that increased fatigue is normal for someone in the Healing Zone. This is true. How tired you feel can be influenced by a variety of factors, including how old you are, what illness or injury you're dealing with, how healthy you were before you became ill, what medications you're taking, what other treatments you're receiving, whether you've been inactive, and how inactive you've become.

That said, it's easy for patients and their doctors to be seduced into thinking that because fatigue is fairly normal during physical recovery, it doesn't require any further investigation. In my opinion, it's best to draw the conclusion that fatigue is "normal" only after checking for and excluding other, potentially treatable causes. Medical reasons for fatigue are extremely common. It's important to not make erroneous assumptions about what's behind low energy. Here's a list of common causes of the fatigue that can affect someone who's in the Healing Zone.

- Alcohol (either excessive consumption or drug-alcohol interactions)
- Anemia
- Anxiety

- Blood sugar (glucose) or hormonal imbalances
- Deconditioning
- Depression
- Infection
- Medical treatments
- Pain
- Prescription or over-the-counter drugs or natural remedies
- Sleep disorders (e.g., sleep apnea)
- Stress (physical or emotional)

Evaluate Your Energy Level during the Day

To help pinpoint the cause of your fatigue, you might begin by considering the following questions.

- Do you feel unusually tired despite sleeping?
- Is sleep restorative for you?
- Are you a restless sleeper?
- Do you have difficulty falling asleep or going back to sleep?
- Do you snore?
- Do you rest or nap during the day?
- Have you curtailed or modified your activities because of your energy level?
- Is fatigue affecting your home life, work, or recreation?
- Do you have difficulty with memory, concentration, attention, or finding the right words to express thoughts?
- Is your energy level considerably different than before you became ill or injured? If so, in what ways?

If you answered yes to two or more of the above questions, then I recommend talking with your doctor about your fatigue. Be sure to ask whether it might be worthwhile to proceed with certain tests to determine (or rule out) a medical explanation for how tired you're feeling.

If you have been taking naps, seriously consider whether they are helping or contributing to your energy crisis. I suggest giving up napping if you are not sleeping well at night. While naps can help make up for a sleep debt in certain circumstances, they also can interfere with your sleep-wake cycle and disrupt your normal sleep patterns. You need to sleep at night to heal optimally, because that's when all those restorative chemical reactions take place. So unless you are convinced that you're better off napping, or if you have another reason to sleep during the day (such as working night shift), try taking a break from it and see whether you notice any improvement in your nighttime sleep and what happens generally to your daytime fatigue.

While napping may be counterproductive, daytime rest is a great idea for everyone, especially those in the Healing Zone. I encourage you to incorporate rest periods into your daily routine—not to sleep but to just relax. See page 48 in Chapter 4 for some suggestions for how to spend your rest breaks so you restore your energy without actually going to sleep.

Cultivate Good Sleep Hygiene

For Super Healing, your long-term goal is fairly straightforward: to regularly obtain at least 8 hours of quality sleep each night and not feel unusually tired during the day. A series of short-term goals may be necessary to help you accomplish this objective. Below, I offer some examples that build on the principles of sleep hygiene. Proper sleep hygiene involves things that you can do at home to promote truly restorative sleep. Just as a number of behaviors can interfere with your ability to fall asleep and stay asleep (e.g., drinking caffeinated beverages late in the day), other behaviors promote relaxation and cultivate a better night's rest (e.g., taking a warm bath or meditating).

Here are the basics of good sleep hygiene.

Manage Your Bedtime Routine

- Go to bed only when you are tired.
- Use your bedroom for sleep and intimacy only (i.e., not to watch television).
- Create a comfortable bedroom environment—moderate temperature, dark, and quiet.
- Try to establish a regular bedtime and wake-up time.
- Develop a bedtime routine that you faithfully follow.
- Plan to get 7 to 8 hours of sleep each night.
- Get rid of your bedroom clock (or hide it if you need the alarm to wake you in the morning).
- If you are unable to fall asleep in about 20 to 30 minutes, get out of bed and go to another room.

Avoid Things That Interfere with Sleep

- Don't eat a heavy meal—especially one high in sugar—before going to bed.
- Avoid drinking a lot of fluids before going to bed.
- Stop drinking caffeine at least 4 to 6 hours before bedtime.
- Eliminate nicotine before bedtime.
- Avoid alcohol after dinner (4 to 6 hours before bedtime).
- Try not to exercise within at least 2 hours of bedtime (some suggest 6 hours).
- Don't watch television or play computer games right before bed.
- Avoid napping during the day.
- Be aware that sleeping pills often are effective only when used for a short period (2 to 4 weeks) and that some sleep aids actually can aggravate a sleep problem.

Relax before Bedtime

- Take a warm bath (not a shower).
- Have a light snack such as a piece of fruit or a bowl of cereal.
- Practice relaxation techniques such as biofeedback, meditation, deep breathing, and imagery.
- Allow at least an hour before bedtime to relax and unwind.

Talk with Your Doctor

Evaluating your daytime energy level and practicing proper sleep hygiene certainly are good starting points for restoring a good night's sleep. But these won't address underlying sleep problems such as sleep apnea or medical issues that contribute to fatigue, such as anemia. Therefore, it's wise for at least one of your short-term goals to be scheduling a visit to your doctor to discuss sleep and fatigue. Talking with someone who knows you and your health status can be very helpful.

Though that may seem like an obvious step, most people don't make an effort to do it. In fact, according to a Gallup poll, 70 percent of Americans who reported experiencing sleep problems said that they never had mentioned it to their doctors. It really is worth doing, especially while you are in the Healing Zone. To facilitate this conversation, I've included a list of the information your doctor will need in order to accurately assess what might be contributing to your fatigue (see "Helpful Information for Your Doctor").

To ensure the best outcome to your conversation, I encourage you to approach the topic of sleep and fatigue in a way that will make clear it's of real concern for you. It isn't easy for physicians who are treating patients with serious injuries and illnesses to focus their attention elsewhere—such as on how to address an underlying sleep disorder. After all, office visits tend to be short, and doctors don't have time to address every issue, so they typically attend to the most critical ones.

Because sleep is so important while you're in the Healing Zone, it's to your advantage to get your doctor to pay attention and really focus on what you're experiencing. You might start your conversation with an opening line like this: "I'm having difficulty sleeping at night, and I feel very tired during the day. I know that some level of fatigue is normal for my situation, but I'd like to talk with you about my symptoms to see if there's anything we can do to help me feel better. In order for you to evaluate this, I brought a list of my symptoms and a list of my current medications, including all of the over-the-counter drugs and supplements I take."

Your doctor may decide to order tests or instruct you to adjust your medication regimen. There are a number of ways in which the two of you can address the dual problem of poor sleep at night and fatigue during the day. Only your doctor can fully evaluate what's best for you.

You might be wondering, "If my doctor doesn't find anything wrong, is it better for me to take a sleeping pill than to not sleep well?" The answer to this question is "probably"—but you and your doctor will need to decide together. There are many more sleep medications available today than in the past. Most of the newer drugs are quite safe, compared with older alternatives such as Valium, which can cause a dependency with long-term use.

On page 118, I've provided a list of the most common sleep aids to give you a sense of your options. Some of these medications are available over the counter, while others require a prescription. I am not endorsing any particular one; it really depends on your specific situation. Your doctor can help determine whether any of them are appropriate for you. While I am not promoting the use of sleep aids generally, I heartily endorse the idea of getting a good night's sleep.

Another Super Healing Synergy

You already are familiar with the Super Healing Synergy that involves getting proper rest, eating to heal, and exercising in a therapeutic manner. There is another Super Healing Synergy, as well as a companion Triple

Helpful Information for Your Doctor

You can help your doctor to really focus on your issues with sleep and fatigue by providing the following information.

- A list of all of the medications you're taking, both prescription and over-the-counter
- A list of any supplements you're taking
- A list of your symptoms (e.g., when you feel tired, whether you snore, how fatigue is affecting your ability to function)
- A description of your mood
- Details about your alcohol and caffeine consumption
- Your sleep schedule (e.g., what time you go to bed, how long it takes you to fall asleep, whether you awaken during the night and why, what time you get up in the morning, whether you nap)
- A description of your activity level during the day

To determine (or rule out) a possible cause of your fatigue, your doctor may recommend one of the following screening tests:

Laboratory Blood Tests

- Complete blood count
- Erythrocyte sedimentation rate
- Creatinine and urea nitrogen
- Glucose
- Calcium and phosphorus
- Electrolytes
- Albumin and total protein
- Liver function
- Thyroid function
- Rheumatology screen
- C-reactive protein
- Viral titers (e.g., Lyme, HIV, Epstein-Barr)

Other Diagnostic Tests

- Urinalysis
- Chest x-ray
- Echocardiogram and/or electrocardiogram
- Sleep study

Sleep Medications

Below are examples of popular sleep aids, both over-the-counter and prescription. You may want to review the list with your doctor to see if one of these medications, or another option, might help you.

Over-the-Counter

- Nytol QuickCaps Caplets
- Simply Sleep Nighttime Sleep Aid Caplets
- Sleepinal Nighttime Sleep Aid Softgels
- Sominex Caplets Maximum Strength
- Tylenol PM
- Unisom Nighttime Sleep Aid SleepTabs
- Unisom SleepGels Maximum Strength

Prescription

- Ambien
- Ambien CR
- Benzodiazepines—e.g., estazolam (ProSom), flurazepam (Dalmane)
- Lunesta
- Rozerem
- Sonata

Other medications may improve sleep as well. For example, muscle relaxants and antidepressants can have sedating effects while also treating underlying muscle spasms or mood disorders, both of which can disrupt sleep.

Some people rely on alcohol as a relaxant and a sleep aid. Alcohol does not do either of these things well. While it may prove relaxing initially, it tends to act as a depressant and affect your mood negatively.

Sleep expert Lawrence Epstein, MD, dispels the myth of alcohol as a sleep aid in *The Harvard Medical School Guide to a Good Night's Sleep*. He calls alcohol the "wolf in sheep's clothing" and cautions that "alcohol is not an effective sleep aid. Its sedative effect may make you fall asleep faster, but it has a harmful effect on sleep quality that far outweighs this benefit."

Threat that can work against optimal physical recovery. It involves a cluster of three symptoms—fatigue, pain, and depressed mood—that can exponentially facilitate recovery or slow healing, depending on whether and how they're managed.

Because each of these symptoms interacts with the other two, if you have an issue with one, then the others are more likely to become troublesome. Likewise, when one improves, so do the others. Although I have devoted a separate chapter to each of these three symptoms, it is important to recognize that they are not completely separate from one another.

You may have noticed that proper rest is a factor in both of the Super Healing Synergies. Recall from the first Super Healing Synergy that you'll be better able to exercise and eat to heal if you sleep well. The same holds true for the second synergy: With adequate good-quality sleep, your mood and pain likely will improve as well.

Any way you look at it, proper rest is paramount. It's important not to underestimate its value in healing.

REMARKABLE RECOVERY

David Rubin

On September 11, 2006, my wife and I were returning to Boston from San Francisco on American Airlines. About two-thirds of the way across the country, my wife happened to look over at me and noticed that I was in distress. My tongue was sticking out and was blue, and my eyes were rolling around in my head. I wasn't aware of any of this. The experience was surreal to me, because I experienced no discomfort, no pain, and no pre–heart attack symptoms whatsoever. I was just sitting next to my wife, reading the newspaper.

The next thing I knew, people were yelling, "Get him on the floor! Get him on the floor!" I was in a sort of la-la land, a dreamlike state, which is about the time I flatlined. I don't know how you would characterize it—maybe the way you might feel just before you fall asleep.

The next thing I remember was people pounding on my chest, and then finally the jolt from the defibrillator that was on the plane, now federally mandated. American Airlines later sent me a printout of the defibrillator, and I could see that I had flatlined for several minutes. I think I probably was dead, but not permanently.

So I was a very lucky guy, number one because my wife looked over at me when she did. The second piece of luck was that I was on an airplane, not driving a car or walking down a street, in which case I probably wouldn't have had a successful resuscitation. And the third piece of luck was that we happened to put down in Milwaukee, of all the places that we could have put down. It was an emergency landing, and I was taken to St. Luke's Medical Center, which is one of the top cardiac facilities in the country.

I was in a brand-new, state-of-the-art 10-story building that was part of the medical center but devoted to nothing but cardiac care. The care that I got there was superb, not only from a surgical point of view in the professionalism of the doctors and nurses, but also in the hospital pre-op and post-op. The people in Wisconsin are wonderful.

I got there at about 8 o'clock in the evening of September 11. On September 12 they did a cardiac catheterization, which indicated that stents were not appropriate and that I would require a double-bypass, open-heart surgical procedure. I had surgery on September 14, and on September 25—11 days later—I was on a plane back to Boston. I have been recuperating since then. I'm the type that sort of fights taking time off because I'm never satisfied with what I'm accomplishing in the day. But I think that appropriate rest and sleep is probably the best healing tool that I can use now.

So as the surgeon in Milwaukee pointed out, it was just a combination of circumstances that made me a very lucky man. He said, "You fell out of the sky into a haystack." I'm very thankful and appreciative of the nurse on the plane who ran up and worked on me, together with a doctor who was on the plane and the flight attendant. I was lucky that I got to St. Luke's Medical Center, and I was lucky that my wife saw me when she did. So there's a great deal of luck involved. Like my dad used to say, to be successful you need a combination of luck and brains, and if you have a choice, take luck.

I had several previous experiences with the health care system. When I was 9 years old I had polio. I felt like I had a 100 percent recovery. I led a very active A-type life—played squash for 25 years, was in the Army Air Corps in World War II, and used to leap tall buildings in a single bound. Then, starting about 8 or 9 years ago, the day after the third arthroscopic surgery on my knee, which comes from all that squash activity, there was a limp.

Since then, in the last 8 years, I've had a progressive weakening in my legs from my waist down due to something called post-polio syndrome. This has been a different kind of experience, because the physical limitations that I am now confronted with are daunting—particularly for somebody who has great difficulty accepting assistance for anything. I also have survived both prostate and lung cancer.

So I'm a very lucky man. I'm 80 years old, and I really do consider myself lucky.

Chapter 8

Alleviate Pain

In order to Super Heal, it's important to alleviate as much pain as possible. There are three primary reasons for doing this.

First, if you are experiencing pain or discomfort, it almost certainly is affecting other aspects of your life—such as how you are sleeping, eating, and exercising. As we discussed in the previous three chapters, this trio of factors is incredibly important to healing well. If pain interferes with any of them, it may set the stage for a suboptimal recovery.

Second, uncontrolled pain can suppress your immune system, as has been demonstrated in both human and animal studies of experimental pain conditions (created via electrical shock, surgery, and other methods). The obvious conclusion, then, is that controlling pain will improve healing. While more research is necessary in this area, the evidence to date is quite convincing that for optimal recovery, alleviating pain is critical.

Third, and arguably the most important, you deserve the best possible quality of life, despite serious illness or injury. The research on how pain undermines quality of life is overwhelming. No one should accept more pain than they need to. There is no doubt that addressing your pain will make your trip through the Healing Zone—and beyond—more pleasant.

Pain as a Constant Companion

One day I was driving with my two daughters in the backseat. They were having an interesting conversation about pain. It went something like this.

> "I have three Band-Aids on my body. One I have on my knee from when I fell down. Another one is from the splinter that Mom had to take out. The third one is where the nurse gave me a shot."

"Oh yeah, well I have a Band-Aid from the shots, too. Plus, I had to have my braces tightened, and that really hurts."

"Well, remember last night I had a headache?"

"I've had a headache before, too!"

And on it went . . .

Pain is a nearly constant companion throughout our lives. All of us have experienced the kinds of painful conditions that my daughters described. These pains, though bothersome, are fleeting and not terribly severe.

Serious illness or injury can involve much more intense, long-lasting pain. It can be from the condition itself, an uncomfortable medical procedure, or medication. Whatever its source, pain is a common occurrence on the journey through the Healing Zone. Trying to completely eliminate it isn't usually possible, nor is it necessarily a good idea.

My knowledge about pain management comes not just from working with patients who have pain conditions but also from experiencing many different kinds of pain myself, especially during my cancer treatment. The two worst kinds were side effects of medication. One was neuropathy, or nerve damage in my hands and feet—the result of a chemotherapy drug that is toxic to nerves. The other was a deep aching in my bones caused by a medication that helped to keep my white blood cell counts from dropping too low. (White blood cells are produced in the bone marrow.)

After I finished the course of these drugs, I found myself dealing with other aches and pains that had much to do with going through such a grueling experience. I developed foot, shoulder, and neck pain—all related to the fact that my body had changed dramatically because of cancer and its treatment.

A Historical Perspective

Pain has been present throughout human history, and doctors long have recognized that any pain symptom is an important clue to the underlying ailment. As Charles Horace Mayo—who with his brother founded the Mayo Clinic—once observed, "Of all the symptoms for which physicians are consulted, pain in one form or another is the most common and often the most urgent. Properly assessed, it stands preeminent among sensory phenomena of disease as a guide to diagnosis."

The word *pain* comes from both the French *peine* and the Latin *poena,* which mean "a penalty or punishment." This etymology reflects the unfortunate historical belief that suffering was divinely imposed as penance for sinful acts. Many people still adhere to this idea, whether consciously or not. When they become ill, they ask themselves, "What have I done to deserve this?"

In 1846—when doctors at Massachusetts General Hospital in Boston first used ether to numb surgical pain—the *People's London Journal* declared, "HAIL HAPPY HOUR! WE HAVE CONQUERED PAIN!" Prior to that, operations were performed with little or no pain relief. Sometimes opium and cannabis were offered out of compassion rather than real efficacy.

Throughout history, humans have resorted to rather remarkable means in an effort to minimize pain and discomfort. The Assyrians, for example, applied pressure on a surgical patient's carotid arteries until he passed out. In 2000 BC, the Chinese were mixing rhododendron and jasmine into a sleeping draft. In the 1500s, army surgeons poured burning oil over gun-shot wounds. Later, they offered the injured a rum-soaked gag or a bullet to bite. Nothing truly worked. Indeed, for surgical patients of the day, there was no alternative to courage.

A famous description of surgery without pain relief comes from a woman named Frances Burney, who wrote of her mastectomy in the early 1800s. Burney described the experience this way.

> When the dreadful steel was plunged into the breast—cutting through veins—arteries—flesh—nerves—I needed no more injunctions not to restrain my cries. I began a scream that lasted unintermittingly during the whole time of the incision—& I almost marvel that it rings not in Ears still . . . so excruciating was the agony.

Though Burney was treated at home, even if she had been hospitalized, her experience likely would have been unchanged. Society held a very different view of pain and suffering in Burney's lifetime than we do today. A snapshot view of hospital practices back then comes from the official "Regulations of the Philadelphia General Hospital," circa 1790. They state:

> Patients may not swear, curse, get drunk, behave rudely or indecently on pain of expulsion after the first admonition. There shall be no card playing or dicing and such patients as are able shall assist in nursing others, washing and ironing linen and cleaning the rooms and such other services as the matron may require.

Saint Augustine declared that the greatest evil is physical pain. Thankfully, over time we have developed many drugs and other therapies to help address this evil. Still, despite significant advances in pain medicine, patients continue to suffer much more than they should. This is why relieving pain, and thus unnecessary suffering, has become such an important component of good health care. In fact, pain has formally been designated the fifth vital sign (after temperature, blood pressure, and heart and respiratory rates). Today, hospitalized patients are not expected to assist with nursing duties—and relieving their pain is paramount to the healing process.

How Pain Interferes with Healing

As mentioned in the previous chapter, pain is one of a cluster of symptoms—the others being depression and fatigue—that commonly occur in the Healing Zone and can prevent optimal recovery. You can turn this Triple Threat into a Super Healing Synergy by finding ways to effectively control each symptom. Remember that addressing any one of these symptoms can lead to improvements in the other two. With this in mind, let's explore the relationships between pain and mood, and pain and sleep, in turn.

Why Pain May Cause Unnecessary Stress and Worry

Studies show that while pain is a physical symptom, it can cause tremendous emotional upheaval. For example, any physical discomfort can cause enormous anxiety in people who have experienced serious heart problems. Worrying about "the next heart attack" is a legitimate concern, though very often the prognosis following surgery is excellent. Moreover, while musculoskeletal pain is common after thoracic surgery, it still can wreak emotional havoc for someone who has experienced a serious heart condition in the past. This kind of worry is present in many other people who have been through serious illness, including cancer.

In my book *After Cancer Treatment: Heal Faster, Better, Stronger,* I describe what I call a pain filter. What often happens in people who have had cancer is that they immediately react to nearly every pain sensation with the thought "Maybe my cancer is back." The brain then needs to filter this thought to evaluate whether it is a legitimate concern.

Though I originally explained how to fine-tune this filter with respect to cancer, the process is just as relevant to many other conditions. Here's what to do.

1. Pain that is new, unidentified, or severe and occurs in the head, chest, or abdomen should be investigated as soon as possible. This type of

physical discomfort may indicate a serious problem that requires immediate medical attention.

2. Pain that is accompanied by other symptoms such as numbness, weakness, or dizziness should be investigated as soon as possible.

3. Physical discomfort after a trauma (e.g., a fall from a ladder or a car accident) should be attended to immediately, regardless of whether there is bleeding or another visible injury.

4. Generally, the pain that people experience is musculoskeletal in origin. This type of discomfort—which commonly affects the neck, low back, and extremities (examples are muscle strains, tendinitis, and osteoarthritis)—tends to not be terribly serious, so the rule of thumb is to wait 2 weeks to see if it disappears on its own. Persistent discomfort should not necessarily alarm you but, rather, prompt you to seek out an appropriate diagnosis and treatment.

5. As you fine-tune your pain filter, remember that serious pain usually declares itself and is hard to ignore. For example, cancer pain typically doesn't wax and wane. Instead, it is the sort of persistent aching that grabs your attention. This is because tumors that grow to the point where they hurt are pressing on structures. Often the pain occurs at night, waking people from sleep.

6. A doctor who can assess the problem and order appropriate tests should evaluate any pain that you experience.

Just as pain can fuel anxiety, anxiety and depression can aggravate pain. It's common for persistent pain and depressed mood to present together in patients. For example, in a study—published in the medical journal *Spine*—of depressive symptoms after a whiplash injury, the researchers found that of approximately 5,000 people, just over 42 percent developed depressive symptoms by 6 weeks postinjury. Another nearly 20 percent exhibited a depressed mood within a year after the whiplash. Not surprisingly, the combination of persistent pain and poor sleep can contribute to depression, too.

How Pain Interferes with Sleep

While it certainly is understandable why people who have survived a heart attack or cancer might fret over any uncomfortable sensations, ignoring pain can slow or impair healing in many other circumstances. I distinctly recall a conversation with a woman who had recently undergone total knee replacement surgery. She said, "If I could just sleep through the night, I could handle the pain during the day." Her words were prophetic of a study that published soon after, in which the researchers noted that while knee replacement was fairly standardized, the outcomes in terms of pain and disability were quite variable. In particular, they determined that higher levels of pain disrupted sleep and predicted poorer functional outcomes 3 months after surgery. The authors concluded, "The present findings underscore the importance of adequate sleep during postsurgical recovery and suggest that interventions targeting sleep disruptions may improve the speed and quality of patients' recovery from [total knee replacement] and other surgical procedures." In other words, pain that interferes with sleep can affect the speed and completeness of recovery.

Studies dating back to the 1930s have shown that sleep deprivation increases pain sensitivity. A more recent study—published in the *Journal of Thoracic and Cardiovascular Surgery* in 2006—found that of more than 500 people who had undergone heart surgery 1 to 3 years earlier, nearly one in four reported chronic pain that was not cardiac in origin (angina). Of those experiencing postoperative pain, almost 40 percent said that it interfered with their general activity level and with sleep. The researchers involved in the study commented, "When patients with and without chronic postoperative pain were compared, the former group had significantly higher levels of anxiety and depression, and they perceived their health-related quality of life as more compromised."

Pain is a factor in many chronic medical conditions. For example, people with diabetes are prone to developing an aching neuropathy in their hands and feet. Recall that sleep problems can interfere with proper glucose metabolism, thus potentially worsening the diabetes itself. Since pain can affect sleep, it stands to reason that people with neuropathy may have sleep issues. This assumption pans out. A study published in the *Clinical Journal of Pain* revealed that people with diabetes and painful neuropathy report significantly worse sleep problems than the general population.

It probably makes sense that pain can affect your ability to achieve a good night's sleep. Even if you don't awaken from the pain, it can cause nighttime restlessness and reduce your sleep quality.

There are several theories about how pain affects sleep. The first is what I just explained—that pain augments nighttime arousals. Another is that pain and sleep share common biological pathways, including the serotonergic system that regulates serotonin and other compounds with an impact on pain, mood, appetite, and so on. A third theory is that poor sleep can interfere with the way in which you process pain—meaning that if you don't sleep well, you become more sensitive to discomfort.

Each of these theories may play a role, or perhaps one is more significant than the others. The answer will be revealed by research over time. What is clear is that pain and sleep have a strong relationship with each other. This is a classic "good news, bad news" situation. The bad news is that pain disrupts sleep, and poor sleep makes us more sensitive to pain. The good news is that improving sleep helps alleviate pain and vice versa.

How to Alleviate Pain

On my bookshelf sits a book called *Management of Pain,* which was penned by a man named John Bonica more than a half century ago. Bonica was born in 1917 in Filicudi, an island off the coast of Sicily. When he was 10 years old, his family moved to the United States, seeking a better life. Five years later, his father died, leaving John in charge of his family. He worked at any job he could find—hawking newspapers, shining shoes, selling fruits and vegetables.

The choice of a career in medicine seemed a stretch for this teenage immigrant from a poor family. Bonica was determined, though. To support himself through school, he took up exhibition wrestling, using the name Johnny Bull or the Masked Marvel. His vocation—which resulted in many injuries—and his medical training gave Bonica a great deal of insight into pain and its treatment.

The late John Bonica, MD, undoubtedly is the most famous pain physician to date. He is the inventor of modern pain clinics that use a multidisciplinary approach, and his classic textbook remains in print (though with new editors). This huge tome, which in its current incarnation runs more than 2,000 pages, is an excellent resource for doctors. Its sheer weight and volume is a reminder of how important treating physical comfort is—and how complicated it can be, since pain is a factor in almost every medical condition.

It would be impossible to distill into a single chapter what Dr. Bonica and his colleagues have detailed in 2,000-plus pages. Nevertheless, there are some tried-and-true ways to approach pain that can help you on your journey through the Healing Zone. The most important points about pain and physical recovery are as follows.

Pain is a symptom that needs to be explored with the goal of getting a proper diagnosis.

Physical discomfort can come from any number of different sources. Trying to identify the source of your pain is critical.

One of my patients—I'll call him Ken—is a polio survivor who has quite a bit of residual paralysis but is able to walk. Though he's only in his late forties, his hip and knee joints have aged prematurely because his muscles aren't strong enough to support his body and protect his joints. One day Ken called my office to request an appointment because his hip was hurting. When I saw him, he told me that I had miraculously cured his pain in the past, and he was hoping for a similar miracle this time.

Ken had already seen his orthopedist, who took an x-ray and told him that he likely would need a hip replacement because the arthritis was severe. When I questioned Ken and then examined him, I came to the conclusion that rather than having the typical arthritic hip pain that radiates to the groin, he had a lateral aching directly over a bursa (a fluid-filled sac that helps protect the hip joint). I told Ken that I thought his symptoms were caused by bursitis rather than arthritis and that a corticosteroid injection would do far more than a hip replacement to alleviate his pain.

Ken agreed to try the injection, which I administered that day. A couple of days later, he sent me an e-mail to confirm that the aching indeed had disappeared. Though Ken is relieved to not have any more hip pain and delighted to not need surgery, his outcome is attributable not to a miracle but, rather, to a simple case of making the right diagnosis.

While you are in the Healing Zone, you may experience significant discomfort from more than one source. It's important to talk with your doctor about your symptoms and accurately explain where you're hurting, what the pain feels like (e.g., sharp or stabbing), how severe it is (you can use a numeric scale in which 10 is intolerable and 0 is no pain at all), when it occurs, what makes it better or worse, and whether it wakes you at night. Also mention any associated symptoms such as numbness or tingling.

As I've mentioned, I always encourage my patients to "listen to the voice of their bodies," which means paying attention to uncomfortable symptoms while at the same time trying not to jump to conclusions that may be inaccurate. In Ken's case, he knew he'd likely have significant arthritis in his hip because of his history of paralysis. The x-ray confirmed the diagnosis. Most people, including many doctors, assume that when they see arthritis, it is the source of discomfort. It can be, but—as with Ken—it isn't always.

It was easy for Ken and his orthopedist to assume that the pain was due to a lack of cartilage in the hip joint. But with a little further investigation and thought, a simple injection proved to be both diagnostic (since the injection alleviated all of the pain, we know that the bursa was the source) and therapeutic.

Pain can be treated in many different ways, and often a combination works best.

Bonica's textbook is huge because so many medical conditions cause physical discomfort and so many treatments can provide relief. In general, pain treatments fall into several categories.

- Conservative pain management is often the first-line approach. By "conservative," we mean that the therapies are not invasive. Examples include (but are not limited to) medications, ice and heat applications, and physical and occupational therapy.

- Integrative therapies typically are not part of mainstream medicine, but they have enough scientific evidence to warrant recommending them in certain situations, such as treating pain. Among the better-known integrative therapies for pain relief are acupuncture and massage.

- Invasive procedures such as injections and surgery are occasionally necessary first-line treatments. In acute appendicitis, for example, surgery is the best choice from the start.

My mother is a very nurturing person who frequently asks me to help out with the various ailments of her friends and acquaintances. Mom has two daughters who are doctors; my sister, Laura, is a pediatrician. We good-naturedly divide her queries into two categories. Laura gets the calls about kids, and I get the calls about adults. I'm always happy to assist if the problem is within my area of expertise, which most types of pain are. Physiatrists often are called pain doctors for this very reason.

On one occasion my mom—a former teacher—asked me to call her friend, a very dear woman who was my sixth-grade teacher. This woman was complaining of an aching shoulder, due to a problem with her rotator cuff. The pain was so severe that she was not leaving her home. She had scheduled an appointment with her doctor for the following week, but she was suffering terribly in the interim. I called her, and in the course of asking a few questions, I learned that she was taking a combination over-the-counter medication with a relatively low dose of two pain relievers—ibuprofen and acetaminophen.

While she was worried that she might need surgery, I reassured her that we could try many other things first. To start, I advised her to take a larger dose of straight ibuprofen three times a day, along with acetaminophen in between doses of the anti-inflammatory. Combination medications often provide too little of any single drug to effectively relieve pain. (See "Common Pain Medications and Their Potential Side Effects" for a list of commonly prescribed pain medications.) Next, I instructed her to ice her

COMMON PAIN MEDICATIONS AND THEIR POTENTIAL SIDE EFFECTS

Many different types of medications can help alleviate pain. Your doctor can assist you in finding the right combination and the proper doses to give you the most relief with the fewest side effects. Here's a rundown of the more common pain medications, along with their possible side effects.

MEDICATION	SIDE EFFECTS*
Acetaminophen	Liver damage
Antidepressants	Sedation, dry mouth, constipation, urinary retention, weight gain
Antiseizure drugs	Dizziness, nausea, blood or liver injury, sedation, weight gain
Lidocaine patch	Skin irritation or rash
Muscle relaxants	Dizziness, sedation, constipation, blood or liver injury
NSAIDs (nonsteroidal anti-inflammatory drugs)	Gastrointestinal bleeding, kidney injury, increased blood pressure
Opiates (narcotics)	Rash/itching, nausea/vomiting, constipation, sedation, dizziness, cognitive impairment, difficulty breathing, urinary retention
Tramadol hydrochloride	Nausea, vomiting, dry mouth, dizziness, sedation

This is not a complete list of side effects.

shoulder for 20 minutes three times a day. Finally, I explained that she may need physical therapy, but she should discuss it with her doctor. Basically, my recommendations boiled down to using several conservative therapies simultaneously to achieve the best results.

A week later, my mom e-mailed me to say that she and her friend—who was feeling much better—went out to dinner and had a wonderful time. Though the woman may need an invasive procedure such as an injection or surgery in the future, for now she's getting significant relief with just the conservative therapies. (To learn more about the available pain injections, see page 132.)

If I were to present all of the options for treating pain, this book would be as large as Bonica's. Here are the broad brushstrokes of several popular conservative and integrative pain therapies.

Medications: As you might imagine, this category includes all of the available pain relievers, both prescription and over the counter. Medications vary greatly both in their chemical composition and in their delivery method—that is, how they're directed to the injured tissue. Usually medications are taken in pill form, though some come as patches, creams, and injections. Two delivery methods for corticosteroids—which can reduce

Common Pain Injections

Injections can be extremely effective for treating localized pain. Delivering the medication directly to injured tissues is easier with a needle than a pill, which must navigate the bloodstream. Here's what is currently available in injectable form.

Botulinum toxin injections: When injected directly into muscles, botulinum toxin reduces muscle spasms, or spasticity. It can help treat the physical effects of spinal cord injury or stroke, as well as the pain of migraine headaches and many other conditions.

Bursitis injections: If the bursa is inflamed, this procedure may involve draining the fluid, followed by injecting medication to reduce inflammation. It may be recommended for conditions such as shoulder and hip bursitis.

Epidural injections: Medication is delivered directly to the epidural space in the spine. It may improve the pain associated with conditions such as spinal stenosis and lumbar/cervical radiculopathy from a bulging disk.

Facet blocks: Injections are administered around the facet joints in the spine to relieve pain usually due to arthritis of the facet joint itself.

Joint injections: Medication is injected into the joint space. It's a common treatment for conditions such as knee arthritis and sacroiliac joint pain.

Nerve blocks: Injections are administered near but not directly into the affected nerve. It may alleviate pain from reflex sympathetic dystrophy (complex regional pain syndrome), carpal tunnel syndrome, and spinal nerve compression syndromes.

Trigger-point injections: They're administered to specific areas of a muscle that generate pain. These injections may reduce muscle spasm and pain in fibromyalgia and other muscle pain syndromes.

Tendon injections: Medication is injected around but not into the tendon to relieve tendinitis.

inflammation over a particular part of your body—are *phonophoresis* and *iontophoresis*. Usually these treatments are administered by a physical or occupational therapist, who applies a corticosteroid onto your skin and then uses a machine to promote its absorption into your skin. Phonophoresis does this via sound waves (similar to ultrasound), while iontophoresis utilizes electrical currents.

Modalities: For pain, the therapeutic modalities include deep heat (such as ultrasound) as well as more superficial heat (hot packs). Cold packs can reduce inflammation and provide a numbing or anesthetic effect. If you use heat or cold therapy at home, be sure to place a towel between the heat or cold source and your bare skin. Remove the heat or cold source after 20 minutes to avoid a burn.

Electrical modalities such as a TENS unit (transcutaneous electrical nerve stimulation) and electrical stimulation—what physical therapists call E-stim—can be helpful. E-stim is performed during a physical therapy session, while a small TENS unit—about the size of a cell phone—can be worn at home.

Exercise: Therapeutic exercise that targets a particular region of the body is great for relieving certain pain conditions. The best way to figure out what will work for you is to enlist the assistance of a physical or occupational therapist. Your doctor can give you an exercise prescription, if she thinks it will be helpful.

Mind-body techniques: These integrative therapies can be terrific at alleviating pain and providing a sense of overall well-being. You can try any number of mind-body techniques that generally are quite safe, including meditation, imagery, biofeedback, and progressive muscle relaxation.

Acupuncture: This is a safe integrative therapy that has proven effective for certain pain conditions. Generally, an acupuncture session is quite comfortable. It takes at least 6 to 8 sessions to see if the treatment is working.

Eliminating all pain is not always a realistic goal for people in the Healing Zone.

Many people wrongly assume that in this day and age, with all of the different options for pain relief, it's possible to eliminate all pain. This simply is not true. Pain almost always is a part of the journey through the Healing Zone, and while alleviating unnecessary physical discomfort is important, making a completely painless journey usually is not realistic or desirable.

There are many reasons for this, but the most important is that pain therapies can have serious side effects, and sometimes the risks of treatment outweigh the benefits. While usually it is very safe to alleviate some discomfort, trying to get rid of all pain can mean that the therapies are too aggressive and the chances of serious side effects too great.

Let's consider opiate (narcotic) medications as an example. Even small doses may affect a person's ability to think clearly and react quickly (which is why their labels caution against driving). In large doses, opiates can impair breathing.

In medicine, such an analysis is known as the risk-benefit profile. In general, the benefit of any given therapy should far outweigh the risks.

Alleviating pain is an important factor in healing.

Despite the fact that it isn't possible to completely alleviate pain, reducing any discomfort will significantly improve your ability to recover optimally. Therefore, as you travel through the Healing Zone, I suggest paying particular attention to this symptom and following the steps in the next section to effectively manage your pain.

For your Super Healing Plan, write out specific goals that focus on relieving discomfort (see "Short- and Long-Term Pain Management Goals" for examples). Remember that when it comes to physical discomfort, toughing it out usually isn't the best way to physically heal. Even if you can handle the pain emotionally, the physical consequences may prevent an optimal recovery.

5 Steps to Treat Your Pain

Since treating pain can get a bit complicated, it might help to approach the problem strategically. Start by following these five steps.

Step 1: Avoid activities that aggravate your pain. You can do a lot to treat your pain at home by avoiding or modifying activities that worsen your symptoms. For example, if you experience hip pain every time you walk or run, switch to another activity such as cycling or swimming, which involves less strain on the hip joint.

Step 2: Get a good night's rest. Sleeping well will help alleviate pain. Your muscles and other tissues need this time to relax and recover. Not sleeping well and staying tense through the night (from a muscular perspective, meaning that your muscles never relax completely) lead to more pain during the day.

Step 3: Obtain the proper diagnosis. It's not uncommon for people who are going through the Healing Zone to accept a higher level of pain or discomfort than they need to. To avoid this, talk with your doctor about your specific pain symptoms and get an accurate diagnosis.

Step 4: Try more than one thing to relieve your pain. As you've seen, there are many options for treating pain. You may need to try more than one and possibly do them simultaneously. Let's say that you take acetaminophen for your pain and it works just a little bit—not enough to make a real difference. Instead of stopping the acetaminophen, you might combine it with massage or acupuncture. If you still have significant pain, maybe your doctor will add another treatment to this regimen. I'm not suggesting that you continuously add more therapies but, rather, that you mix and match until you find the combination that works for you.

Step 5: Don't get behind the pain. If you wait too long to address the pain, it's going to be more resistant to treatment and more difficult to alleviate. For example, if you wait until you have a full-blown raging headache

Short- and Long-Term Pain Management Goals

Below are several examples of goals that might help you in your efforts to better control your pain. Read through these, then use them as reference points for creating your own goals.

Short-Term

- Keep track of your pain for a month. Note when it occurs, how severe it is, and what makes it better or worse.

- Make an appointment with your doctor specifically to discuss your pain issues and how to manage them.

- Try a few sessions of acupuncture or massage—one session per week.

- If you're using pain medication, ask your doctor whether you can take it earlier in the day to stay ahead of the pain.

- If you tend to be too active or if your pain gets worse with a lot of activity, set aside time every day to take a break and rest.

- Try applying a hot or cold pack for 20 minutes every day to see if it helps.

Long-Term

- Consider scheduling a consultation with a doctor who specializes in treating pain.

- Exercise most days of the week, and include both aerobic conditioning and strength training in your workouts.

- If sleep or mood is an issue, take specific steps to address it.

- If your doctor orders physical therapy or other treatment, follow through with the recommendation.

to take acetaminophen, it might not work. But if you take the medication at the first sign of pain, you might be able to keep the pain from getting worse—or even eliminate it altogether.

Be aggressive about treating your pain early in the day, and you will be better able to control it with less medication and other therapies. Anything you do to treat pain will work better the less pain you have.

Chapter 9

Use Your Mind to Heal Your Body

Telling someone to simply think about healing and it will happen may sound like magic or sorcery. But the mind-body connection isn't just a clever illusion. What you think and feel really does elicit physical responses from your body. In this way, it can affect how you heal.

For example, you probably have heard that psychological factors such as stress play an important role in heart disease. Convincing research has shown that reducing emotional stress can in turn lower the risk of experiencing future heart problems. Though much of the evidence in support of mind-body interventions focuses on heart disease rather than other conditions, it nevertheless offers compelling scientific proof that what's on your mind can help you mend as you travel through the Healing Zone.

The next three chapters will explore what has come to be known as mind-body medicine and its role in physical healing. I'll explain the relationships among mood, love, and spirituality and how each contributes to optimal physical recovery.

The Reemergence of Mind-Body Medicine

It's interesting to trace the idea of an inexorable link between mind and body back to ancient times. In fact, except for the past 300 or so years, scientists and philosophers throughout history were quick to acknowledge this relationship.

The great 15th-century French mathematician and philosopher Rene Descartes, who has been called the father of modern philosophy, wrote of *res extensa* (the bodily function) and *res cogitans* (the function of the soul). Thirty years after Descartes's death in 1650, Hungarian physician Pápai

Páriz Ferenc ascribed to the long-held belief that an imbalance of the mind will lead to an imbalance of the body and vice versa. He offered the following point of view, which was quite common back then.

> When the parts of the body and its humors are not in harmony, then the mind is unbalanced and melancholy ensues, but on the other hand, a quiet and happy mind makes the whole body healthy.

During Ferenc's lifetime, the popular theory was that bodily fluids—called humors—were responsible for physical health. Hence, when the humors were not in balance, people became ill.

Ironically, medicine moved away from treating the mind and body as a whole during the period in the 18th century known as the Enlightenment. At that time, infectious disease was the main threat to existence. In European society of the mid-19th century, only the well-to-do gentry class had access to doctors—not that it mattered much, as there was little these medicine men could really do. Without the sanitation or the medical treatments that are available today, the life expectancy for the English gentry was 43 years. For laborers, it was a mere 23 years.

The advent of vaccines to prevent infections and antibiotics to cure them paved the way for people to view sickness as something that could be overcome with a "magic bullet." It became easy to ignore any relationship between the mind and body. Mainstream Western medicine tended to do just that.

But just as smallpox, tuberculosis, cholera, polio, and other infectious diseases came under control, a new set of health threats began to emerge. These conditions—such as heart disease, high blood pressure, diabetes, and cancer—develop not because of a virus or bacteria but, rather, because of genetic predisposition, lifestyle influences, and/or psychological factors (e.g., stress). With this new set of health threats, doctors and scientists once again began to embrace the idea of an intrinsic connection between mind and body.

Among the modern-day pioneers in mind-body medicine is Herbert Benson, MD, a cardiologist who founded what is now known as the Benson-Henry Institute for Mind Body Medicine at Massachusetts General Hospital. Dr. Benson has conducted many studies to verify how our brains can influence our bodies. He is highly respected and internationally renowned, and his work has helped drive a major philosophical shift within the scientific community about the importance of mind-body medicine in preventing and recovering from serious illness.

Still, this area of medicine remains in its infancy, and it often invites debate. Currently, perhaps the most controversial topic in mind-body medicine is how spirituality influences healing. I'll explore this topic in more detail in Chapter 12. For now, I'll say that the controversy isn't about Dr. Benson's rigorous scientific studies per se but, rather, about spirituality's place in medical practice. It's hard to imagine a time when this topic won't lend itself to intense disagreement. As you read this book, I would encourage you to keep an open mind and focus on the science behind mind-body medicine, which has explored the relationship between spirituality and healing. As Dr. Benson observes, "a belief in God dispatched by our brains is deeply soothing to our bodies."

Dr. Benson may be best known for his work on what he has called the "relaxation response," which is very similar to some forms of meditation. Few people who have studied the relaxation response would question its effectiveness. It is the opposite of the stress response commonly known as fight-or-flight.

Your nervous system has two components: the sympathetic and the parasympathetic. In a stressful situation, the sympathetic nervous system steps up and actually goes into overdrive—increasing your heart rate, breathing rate, blood pressure, and blood circulation in order for your body to react to a stressor. The relaxation response is the exact opposite. It prompts the parasympathetic nervous system to take over, slowing your heart and breathing rates and lowering your blood pressure so that you relax.

Dr. Benson's research has shown that the relaxation response produces measurable and consistent physical changes, including declines in heart and breathing rates, blood pressure, metabolism, and muscle tension and increases in certain brain waves. There is an indisputable mind-body "chain reaction" that takes place when people are able to perform the relaxation response.

The Next Frontier in Healing

Dr. Benson is not alone in trying to rigorously study the relationship between how we function physically and how we function emotionally. In fact, a group of well-respected scientists began to examine this relationship in earnest during the latter part of the 20th century, pioneering a new field of medicine called *psychoneuroimmunology*. This area of research focuses on how our brains and bodies interact and how this interaction influences health and disease.

Dr. Benson and others who have dedicated their careers to mind-body medicine have done so at great risk to their reputations. Their courage and conviction have paid off. Today few people would argue that the mind-body connection is all hooey. Science writer Henry Dreher sums it up this way: "These explorers, leaders of such fields as psychoneuroimmunology, neuroimmunomodulation, and psychoneuroendocrinology, sneaked past the closed doors of biomedical compartmentalization with the fearlessness of cat burglars."

As Dreher explains in his book *Mind-Body Unity*, one reason these "visionary mind-body scientists" have faced so many public opinion obstacles is that mind-body medicine often has been reduced to the simplistic and quite detrimental slogan of "mind over matter." Dreher writes:

> Popular culture has enshrined the concept of a "mind-body connection," . . . [a] term [that] reflects outdated ideas from the predecessor field of psychosomatic medicine, as well as rather simplified concepts that stem from today's broader culture of alternative medicine, a culture that often peddles a one-dimensional "mind over matter" approach to mind-body medicine. (It is generally agreed among mind-body scientists that mind does not lord its putative powers over matter; rather, mind and matter are intertwined in a kind of dialectic dance.)

Currently, much of the research in the mind-body field is focusing on the physical effects of therapies such as meditation, imagery, prayer, relaxation, biofeedback, and hypnosis. Though it is absolutely clear that our brains affect our bodies in numerous ways (and vice versa), it is not a linear relationship for which there is a straightforward cause-and-effect outcome.

Though we have learned a lot about the mind-body relationship, including how stress affects us, much remains for us to discover. As the research continues, old ideas—such as the belief that all stress is harmful and results in depressed immune function—gives way to a better understanding of how stress can be helpful in some instances and harmful in others (depending on factors such as how long the stress lasts, how severe it is, and how well prepared we are to handle it). The bottom line is that in this field of medicine, while we know for certain that the mind-body flow is bidirectional, simple platitudes such as "all stress is bad" no longer seem to hold up.

Although we don't fully understand all of the intricacies of mind-body medicine, we know enough to use mind-body therapies to help with physical healing. Deepak Chopra, MD, an endocrinologist by training and a leader in the field of mind-body medicine, has suggested that some people are "geniuses of the mind-body connection." Dr. Chopra believes that those who can tap into the enormous potential of the mind-body relationship are capable of what he calls "quantum healing."

Snake-Oil Salesmen versus HMO Executives

If you are a bit skeptical about mind-body therapies, you are right to be so. Mind-body therapies fall into the category of complementary and alternative medicine (CAM). CAM encompasses treatments that typically are outside of mainstream medicine. In the past, few CAM therapies were subject to rigorous scientific study, and fewer still proved their efficacy. Recently, however, many more scientists have been turning an eye toward these treatments. The ones that have shown themselves to be beneficial in scientific studies now are known as *integrative therapies*. Doctors formally prescribe these treatments, usually in combination with conventional medical measures.

Many CAM therapies still have not undergone rigorous scientific study. This doesn't mean that they don't work; it just means that they lack the evidence to offer them alongside mainstream treatments that have stood up to scientific scrutiny. Unfortunately, lumped in with many legitimate and respectable CAM practitioners are the charlatans and snake-oil salesmen who prey on those who are ill and vulnerable—often cheating them out of hard-earned money and, even more important, causing a delay in treatment that can make a tremendous difference in how well someone heals.

Not surprisingly, some people are ardent believers in CAM therapies and go to extraordinary lengths to pursue them. At the other end of the spectrum are those who uniformly dismiss anything that smacks of alternative medicine. Journalist Steve Salerno is extremely skeptical of CAM therapies; his book *Sham: How the Self-Help Movement Made America Helpless* is a rather harsh critique of the CAM industry. Salerno characterizes the mind-set of those who relentlessly pursue alternative therapies this way: "The alt-med mind-set thus promotes a bizarre, inverse credibility wherein the further something strays from mainstream approval, the more cachet it achieves among alt-med subscribers."

The CAM industry is enormous in industrialized countries, and you don't have to be dumb to be duped by it. One of my patients, whom I'll call Bill, is a high-level executive at a company that you would easily recognize. As vice president and chief financial officer, Bill travels throughout the world on a regular basis. Three years before coming to see me, he developed low back pain. It was manageable at first, but as it became more severe, Bill began to seek out treatment. Unfortunately, this highly intelligent individual completely opted out of conventional medicine and instead turned to CAM. He tried massage therapy, acupuncture, naturopathic medicine, and chiropractic treatment—all without any relief.

After investing 3 years and thousands of dollars in CAM treatments, Bill limped into my office. His pain was so intense that he no longer was able to travel. He even had difficulty performing his day-to-day duties at the office. This "numbers guy"—who one would think would want the benefit of scientific evidence behind his treatment—hadn't even gone to a medical doctor for an exam. Thus, he'd not had what we in mainstream medicine would consider an appropriate work-up.

Because Bill's pain radiated from his low back down his leg and was associated with nervelike symptoms such as numbness, tingling, and leg weakness, I ordered a magnetic resonance imaging (MRI) study of his low back. This very reliable, state-of-the-art study confirmed what I suspected: A herniated disk was crushing one of his nerve roots. The protruding disk was large, and Bill was quite physically compromised by the pain and leg weakness. (Because nerves feed into muscles, an injury to a nerve can result in paralysis of the muscles.)

I advised Bill to go for a surgical consultation. As the surgeon explained, none of the alternative therapies that Bill had tried would work for his particular health situation. Studies had shown that he likely would experience the best outcome if he opted for an operation. While not all disk herniations require surgery, when a significant nerve injury results in partial paralysis of the muscles, an operation can offer the best chance of alleviating pain and regaining strength.

Bill was at a loss for words when I asked him to explain why he stayed with a completely alternative medical regimen for such an inordinately long time when it clearly wasn't working. I still don't know why he did what he did, and I suspect that he doesn't, either. There probably are several reasons. First, he relied on the advice of family, friends, and alternative practitioners rather than a medical doctor to guide his treatment. Second, with his busy schedule, it was easier and more convenient for him to schedule appointments for CAM therapy. Finally, like a lot of people, Bill didn't think all that highly of medical doctors, who always seemed a bit rushed and not all that concerned about him—unlike the CAM practitioners, who were willing to spend time with him. (Studies show that people really appreciate the time and attention that they get from CAM practitioners, which can translate into a confidence level in their healing abilities that may not be warranted.)

Do I seem to be contradicting myself? On the one hand, I am saying that the mind-body relationship is extremely important, while on the other hand, I am suggesting that conventional "body-oriented" medicine is the way to go. Both statements are true, and there is some middle ground between the two. This is where the phrase "complementary medicine" comes into play. A mind-body therapy qualifies as complementary medicine when it is used in conjunction with—not instead of—conventional medicine. If the therapy falls into the integrative medicine category, it's even better, because it means that the therapy has been studied and deemed appropriately safe and beneficial.

Conventional medicine has a lot to offer. As you'll recall from Chapter 2, on your journey through the Healing Zone, your conductor should be a medical doctor who is knowledgeable of the latest research and the best treatments for your condition. This is why I don't recommend utilizing CAM therapies or an alternative approach exclusively. Instead, aim for a complementary or, better yet, an integrative approach for the quickest and safest journey through the Healing Zone.

While some CAM providers are charlatans, even the most die-hard conventional medicine devotees have to admit that certain mind-body treatments can help keep disease from occurring and support healing when it does. It isn't surprising that HMO administrators are among the most reticent to fully embrace mind-body therapies. These folks have the unenviable task of keeping down costs, and one way to do it is to make sure that patients don't get unnecessary treatment—such as therapies that haven't been proven to work.

Interestingly, in a 1997 survey of HMO executives, 90 percent of respondents indicated that they believe personal prayer, meditation, or religious practices can support medical treatment and potentially expedite the healing process. The same survey also revealed that 90 percent of these executives want to see more scientific evidence before agreeing to cover these services. Fortunately, the research confirming the efficacy of certain mind-body therapies has been quite impressive. Because of this, two of three HMOs now provide some coverage for CAM therapies, such as spiritual counseling, that fall within their integrative medicine program. As the textbook *Integrative Medicine: Principles for Practice* summarizes:

> Mind-body medicine—the interplay of mind, emotions, and physical processes in health and illness—encompasses a philosophy of care, a body of research, and approach to therapy . . . characterized by a philosophical commitment to whole-person care. Its origins are found in ancient and holistic healing traditions, which strive for unity of mind, body, and spirit . . . The mind-body connection has been documented by 30 years of laboratory, epidemiologic, and evidence-based clinical research.

The Mind-Body Therapies

There is no question of the existence of a powerful mind-body relationship. Though we don't fully understand it, we can still take advantage of therapies that exploit these healing forces. To me, it's a "best of both worlds" scenario, combining mind-body therapies with conventional medicine to achieve optimal healing.

As you develop your mind-body goals for your Super Healing Plan, I suggest trying one of the following therapies: meditation, imagery, or progressive muscle relaxation. All are safe and easy to do, though you don't need to practice all of them. Start with the one that feels most comfortable for you and work from there. Let's look at each technique in turn. (To see how you might build your goals around these techniques, see page 144.)

Meditation

Of the three therapies that I mention above, meditation is the one most supported by research. Meditation takes many forms, the majority of which originated as ancient religious or spiritual practices. But you can meditate in a way that is completely secular.

The basic idea behind meditation is to relax your mind and body. It likely works in part by promoting the parasympathetic nervous system response, slowing your heart and breathing rates as well as lowering your blood pressure.

Scientific studies that used a special brain imaging technique called functional magnetic resonance imaging (fMRI) have shown that when people meditate, a number of physical changes occur simultaneously. In one such study, meditation increased activity in the left side of the brain, toward the front. Not surprisingly, this is the same area that regulates positive emotions. In the same study, people who meditated showed elevated blood levels of certain immune chemicals. The researchers concluded that meditation likely not only improves mood but also can boost the immune system.

Meditating is easy to learn, though it does take practice. You'll get better and better at it the more you do it. Many books, tapes, CDs, and DVDs can guide you through a meditation session. If you'd rather try it on your own, here's all you need to do.

1. Find a quiet location.
2. Sit or lie down comfortably.
3. Focus your attention on something—your breath, a word or phrase, or an object.
4. Keep an open mind, and let distractions come and go without stopping to think about them.

As you're starting out, try meditating for just a few minutes. Increase your time as you get comfortable with the technique.

Short- and Long-Term Mind-Body Goals

The following examples of short- and long-term goals will show you how you might go about incorporating mind-body techniques into your Super Healing Plan.

Short-Term

- Spend 5 minutes a day meditating. Set the kitchen timer and stop when it goes off.
- Read a book on how to meditate.
- Listen to a meditation CD or tape twice a week and follow along with it.
- Spend 5 minutes a day practicing imagery.
- Read a book on imagery.
- Listen to an imagery CD or tape twice a week and follow along with it.
- Perform progressive muscle relaxation once a day.

Long-Term

- Meditate twice a day for up to 30 minutes at a time.
- Practice imagery twice a day.
- Perform progressive muscle relaxation twice a day.

Imagery

As its name suggests, imagery involves using your mind to develop a mental image of something. The theory is that the mind is able to cure the body when a particular mental image evokes sensory memory, strong emotions, or fantasy.

One of my favorite images is from a painted card that an artist friend and cancer survivor sent me. On the front is a picture of a tree—but if you look closely, you see that the tree is also a woman. The two images are meshed together. On the back of the card my friend wrote, "Strong as a tree—and reaching up—up to faith and surrounded by those who love her."

Another image that I used during my cancer treatment was one that a fellow doctor and cancer survivor had suggested. She told me to imagine a day in the future when I'm at my daughter's wedding and to "see" all of the details of what will be a wonderful occasion.

You can use any image you find appealing; in fact, you can change images each time you practice this technique. The point is to promote positive thoughts and encourage your parasympathetic nervous system to slow your heart and breathing rates and lower your blood pressure.

Progressive Muscle Relaxation

Progressive muscle relaxation involves tensing and then relaxing all of the muscles throughout your body in sequence. Sit or lie down in a comfortable place. Working from head to toe, start by grimacing and clenching your teeth for a count of 10. Then relax, inhaling and exhaling as you do. Let your face be as lax as if you were asleep. Next, tense the muscles in your neck and shoulders for a count of 10; relax. Repeat, using the muscles in your chest, abdomen, buttocks, arms, hands, legs, and feet.

Thoughts on Healing

In the 1970s—before the field of psychoneuroimmunology had become well established—Norman Cousins, MD, wrote a now-famous book titled *Anatomy of an Illness as Perceived by the Patient*. In this book, Dr. Cousins discussed many aspects of mind-body medicine and how they may affect health. He summarized the mind-body relationship with these words: "What we are talking about essentially . . . is the chemistry of the will to live."

Dr. Cousins had little evidence to support his claims; not surprisingly, some experts regarded his book with a fair amount of skepticism. More than 2 decades later, Larry Dossey, MD, would reinforce Dr. Cousins's sentiment: "Today almost everyone recognizes the role of emotional stress in heart disease; that depression can inhibit our body's immune function; and that people who attend to their mental health—their satisfaction, joy, and fulfillment—generally live longer and are healthier than people who do not."

Indeed, a large and growing body of research confirms what Dr. Cousins first theorized decades ago. I would venture to say that mind-body medicine is not only a life force but also a healing force that can assist people in recovering from serious illness and injury.

Chapter 10

Monitor Your Mood

In this chapter, we'll focus on how your mood can affect your ability to heal optimally. I am not suggesting that you need to be happy all the time. That would be impossible, even under the best circumstances. But I am hoping that you'll consider how your thoughts engage certain areas of your brain that in turn trigger certain physiological responses in your body. In other words, you can use your mind to promote physical healing. Your emotional state is part of this equation.

Stress, Health, and Healing

Whenever people ask me about stress, I always tell them that an important part of healing is finding ways to relax. At the same time, I encourage them not to add to their burden by worrying about worrying.

Psychological stress affects you physically through a very complex set of chemical reactions. The process begins with a trigger, which can be either acute (meaning sudden, such as a car accident) or chronic (for example, a difficult work situation). The brain responds to the trigger by activating several of the body's systems, including the immune, endocrine, and nervous systems. They in turn release various compounds that alter the chemical reactions taking place in the body. These compounds—which have been measured in research studies on stress—include cortisol, prolactin, substance P, nerve growth factor, and corticotropin-releasing hormone.

Literally thousands of studies have examined the physiological effects of stress. Much of this research has focused on the link between stress and heart attacks and leaves no doubt that stress contributes to cardiac vulnerability. Among the key findings to date:

- Emotional stress elevates both blood pressure and heart rate.

- More heart attacks occur on Mondays than on any other day of the week.

- An increase in the number of heart attacks occurs on two major holidays: Christmas and New Year's.

- The number of heart attacks also rises after a major disaster (such as an earthquake).

- In one study, people were six times more likely to have a heart attack if they were facing a high-pressure deadline at work.

A significant number of studies also have explored how stress affects immune function and healing. Some of the highlights:

- People under stress are more susceptible to upper respiratory infections.

- Stress increases interleukin-6, a factor in the body's inflammatory response.

- Stress tends to decrease the activity of immune cells known as natural killer cells.

- People with post-traumatic stress disorder have higher levels of stress hormones called catecholamines (e.g., norepinephrine, epinephrine, and dopamine).

- In healthy people, chronic sleep deprivation—which causes both emotional and physical stress—raises blood pressure, blood glucose, insulin, cortisol, and proinflammatory cytokines.

Richard Cohen knows a lot about stress. He was just 25 years old when he learned that he had multiple sclerosis. Thirty years later, he fought colon cancer twice in the same year. Though he may be best known as the husband of Meredith Vieira, coanchor of NBC's *Today* show, he is an extremely talented man in his own right. Cohen's list of accomplishments includes stints as a senior producer for CBS News and CNN. He also is a three-time Emmy Award winner.

In his poignant memoir *Blindsided: Lifting a Life Above Illness,* Cohen—in a manner consistent with his television news background—writes about himself with both an objective detachment and a passion that helps readers understand that while illness has taken its toll on his body, he is determined to live life to the fullest extent possible. Cohen avoids the Pollyannaish tendency of some writers to glorify illness and instead shares how he really feels. At one point, he tells readers, "Anger is my unyielding, live-in companion, though I have tried to break up that relationship for years." He is acutely aware that while he can't completely control his emotions, he needs to try. As he writes, "Citizens of sickness, those who suffer from their own assaults on body and spirit, know disappointment. . . . The battle to control our heads is every bit as important as combating the attacks on our bodies."

Why Mood Matters

There is no question that when it comes to physical healing, mood matters. Before we delve too far into this subject, let's explore *why* mood matters. Test your psychological health acumen by answering the following true-or-false questions.

1. Mood is important to physical healing primarily because it can help motivate someone to focus on recovery.

2. Mood is something you almost always can control.

3. For optimal healing, you need to avoid negative emotions such as anger, sadness, worry, and grief.

If you answered false to each of these questions, you're absolutely right. These are what I call Mood Myths, and it's helpful to dispel them up front. Now let's move on to the emotional truisms, or what I call Mood Maxims.

1. Your mood specifically influences chemicals in your body that have a direct effect on physical healing.

2. It is impossible to perfectly control your mood, especially while you are in the Healing Zone and are experiencing so much, both physically and emotionally.

3. Negative emotions are an inevitable part of your journey through the Healing Zone. Though an abundance of them can hamper physical recovery, you can use them to your advantage to help focus on Super Healing.

We'll explore each of these Mood Maxims in greater detail, beginning with the first one.

Emotions Cause Physical Changes in Your Body

Mood Maxim #1: Your mood specifically influences chemicals in your body that have a direct effect on physical healing.

Though the relationship between our emotions and our bodies is as old as mankind, only recently have scientists begun to explore it in earnest. The research to date is compelling, and, as I mentioned in the last chapter, it has led to the establishment of a new field in medicine called psychoneuroimmunology.

As the name suggests, psychoneuroimmunology is the study of how what we experience psychologically affects us physically—especially the brain and the nervous and immune systems. This is a fascinating area of research, with compelling and often surprising insights into how stress and other emotions influence physical healing. Stress, which all of us experience to some degree every day of our lives, is a reliable predictor of delayed wound healing. It also seems to age the body prematurely.

As I mentioned earlier, much of the research about the relationship between mind and body has concentrated on how our emotions, especially stress, can harm our hearts and blood vessels. Cardiologists have known about the deleterious role of stress in heart disease for decades. Richard Helfant, MD, a Harvard-trained cardiologist, describes the cascading effect of stress in his book *Courageous Confrontations*.

> Evidence has now made clear that mental distress increases blood pressure, constricts blood vessels, and increases the tendency of circulating platelets to form clots. When patients are stressed by performing difficult mental tasks in a laboratory setting, the identical circulatory responses can readily be elicited. Mental stress also causes sizeable deterioration in the cardiac function of patients with coronary artery disease.
>
> It has become a cliché that depression is bad for our health, but only recently have effects been scientifically studied. In a recent report, depression was shown to rival high cholesterol as a risk factor for coronary artery disease and heart attacks. Depression affects the circulation through mechanisms similar to those of stress.
>
> Heart attacks usually occur during the early morning hours, when adrenalin and other stress hormones, as well as factors that cause clotting, are at peak activity. Surveys have found that 75 percent of working people dread getting up in the morning.
>
> This dread is particularly intense on Monday mornings. The so-called "Monday morning blues" refers to a time when apprehension about having to confront the stress of the long week ahead is at its peak. Most heart attacks occur on Monday.

Evidence abounds that stress plays a significant role in health and disease. This is a book about physical healing, however, so germane to the topic at hand is the question, how does stress affect physical recovery?

The short answer is that stress slows healing, and the research in this regard is both intriguing and compelling. I'll share just a few of the highlights here.

A now-classic study from 1998 on stress and wound healing involved a group of healthy dental students who had wounds placed in their mouths on two occasions. For the first round, the wounds were timed to coincide with summer vacation. The second round occurred 3 days before the first major academic exam of the term. Not surprisingly, the wounds planted before the exam took 40 percent longer to heal. The researchers concluded, "These data suggest that even something as transient, predictable, and relatively benign as examination stress can have significant consequences for wound healing."

A separate study published in the *British Medical Journal* looked at whether relieving stress would facilitate healing. This time, a group of healthy volunteers received a similar wound in the upper arm using a special research device. The 36 volunteers were divided into two groups. One group was instructed to write about an emotional event in their lives, preferably one they had not talked about much before. The other group wrote about trivial matters. The participants who wrote about emotional events healed faster, leading the researchers to conclude that relieving stress by writing about it is helpful for physical recovery.

Both of these studies involved healthy volunteers and superficial wounds. More recently, researchers have been looking into the relationship between stress and wound healing in people recovering from surgical incisions. One study that appeared in *Psychosomatic Medicine* evaluated psychological stress and wound healing in people recovering from a hernia repair. The researchers concluded that "greater worry" predicted lower levels of matrix metalloproteinase-9 in wound fluid, more pain, and delayed healing. (Matrix metalloproteinase-9 is a protein that facilitates tissue regeneration and healing.)

The findings of these studies certainly help make the case for a strong link between emotions and healing.

You Can't Have Perfect Control over Your Emotions

Mood Maxim #2: It is impossible to perfectly control your mood, especially while you are in the Healing Zone and are experiencing so much, both physically and emotionally.

Though the scientific evidence clearly shows that mood matters to physical healing, it's unrealistic to believe that we can rein in our feelings at such an emotionally charged time in our lives. Nor should we.

Bad moods, grief, and worry are part and parcel of the journey through the Healing Zone. They do need to be tempered with periods of optimism and hope. Having traveled through the Healing Zone myself, I know this may sound easier than it actually is. Serious illness or injury never is what any of us planned for. But as mythologist Joseph Campbell encouraged, "We must be willing to get rid of the life we have planned, so as to have the life that is waiting for us."

Generally, the kinds of day-to-day emotional fluctuations that occur with illness or injury don't require medical attention. That said, it is not uncommon for people who are physically recovering to experience more profound emotional states such as clinical depression, anxiety, or even post-traumatic stress disorder. These require professional care, which may include counseling and perhaps antidepressants or other medications.

The following lists identify the symptoms of emotional issues that may require medical intervention. If you're experiencing any of these symptoms, please talk with your doctor about them as soon as possible.

DEPRESSION: SIGNS AND SYMPTOMS

☐ Losing interest in usual activities and pastimes

☐ Feeling irritable

☐ Crying frequently

☐ Feeling sad

☐ Feeling hopeless

☐ Having a poor appetite or significant weight loss

☐ Having an increased appetite or significant weight gain

☐ Sleeping poorly

☐ Sleeping too much

☐ Feeling agitated or restless

☐ Feeling unusually fatigued

☐ Having difficulty concentrating

☐ Having difficulty making decisions

☐ Feeling self-critical

☐ Feeling excessively guilty

☐ Feeling worthless

☐ Having recurrent thoughts of dying or suicide

ANXIETY: SIGNS AND SYMPTOMS

☐ Feeling tense or nervous

☐ Feeling jittery or jumpy

☐ Having difficulty relaxing

☐ Feeling fatigued

☐ Having muscle aches

☐ Feeling restless

☐ Feeling apprehensive

☐ Feeling fearful or anticipating misfortune

☐ Feeling sweaty or having clammy hands

☐ Having chest palpitations or a racing heart

☐ Having a stomachache

☐ Feeling light-headed or dizzy

☐ Having difficulty sleeping

☐ Feeling "on edge"

☐ Feeling terrified without apparent reason

☐ Anticipating impending doom

☐ Feeling short of breath

☐ Experiencing a choking or smothering sensation

☐ Feeling faint

☐ Trembling or shaking

POST-TRAUMATIC STRESS DISORDER: SIGNS AND SYMPTOMS

☐ Having mental flashbacks

☐ Being startled by loud noises

☐ Feeling anxious or depressed

☐ Sleeping poorly

☐ Having difficulty concentrating

☐ Having nightmares

☐ Feeling irritable

☐ Feeling angry

Taking Time to Grieve

With any trauma or a new diagnosis such as cancer, people often experience a period of shock followed by grief. In his book *Good Grief,* the late

Lutheran pastor and former University of Chicago medicine and religion professor Granger Westberg wrote:

> God has so made us that we can somehow bear pain and sorrow and even tragedy. However, when the sorrow is overwhelming, we are sometimes temporarily anesthetized in response to a tragic experience. We are grateful for this temporary anesthesia, for it keeps us from having to face grim reality all at once.

I'll never forget a young woman I treated while working at a military hospital during my residency. In a fit of anger, fueled by alcohol, this soldier got behind the wheel of a car and ended up colliding with a tree while driving at high speed. Thankfully, she survived this horrific accident, but her arm was so severely injured that it had to be amputated. The young doctors I was working with at the time were amazed at how accepting she seemed of such a disfiguring and disabling injury. The older physicians, our mentors and teachers, wisely advised us that there would undoubtedly come a time when she would fiercely grieve. They were right.

What we saw initially—and it lasted for weeks—was a period of shock during which the young woman was emotionally "anesthetized." She never cried and never appeared sad. Later, she did grieve, crying out with hard, racking sobs that everyone around her could hear. Although it was painful to watch, I am sure that she needed to mourn her arm and her altered life.

It is not uncommon for people to try to avoid mourning a loss, especially if it's a personal loss such as one that can occur with illness or injury. Some people view grieving about themselves as an act of selfishness, though it certainly is not. Others who are deeply religious may deem grieving as akin to having a lack of faith. Westberg addressed this concern in his book.

> Faith plays a major role in grief of any kind. But not in the way some people think. They often seem to have the idea that a person with strong faith does not grieve and is above this sort of thing. Moreover, these people imply that religious faith advocates stoicism. They might even quote the two words from Scripture, "Grieve not!" They forget to quote the rest of the phrase in which these two words are found: "Grieve not as those who have no hope" (1 Thess. 4:13).

Sociology professor and writer Arthur Frank has experienced life-threatening illness twice—once when he had a heart attack at age 39 and the other just months later, when he was diagnosed with testicular cancer. His reflections on illness include these thoughts on mourning.

> These losses of future and past, of place and innocence, whether they are ours together or mine alone, must all be mourned. The ill person's losses vary according to one's life and illnesses. We should never question what a person chooses to mourn. One person's losses may seem eccentric to another, but the loss is real enough, and that reality deserves to be honored.

Sifting through Emotions

There's a storybook that I read to my children about a girl bear whose world is colorful and happy. The book pages depict this cheerful view of her surroundings. Seeing that she is not a cautious bear, however, her mother tells her that the world is filled with strangers and she mustn't talk to them. Suddenly, her worldview changes—and the pages, depicting exactly what happens in the story, become darker and more menacing.

I often thought of this book during my illness. I longed for the bright, lighthearted world that I had inhabited, but the one I was in was much darker and more frightening—at least for a time. By the end of the story, the young bear has more perspective. Though her world has changed a bit, it still is a wonderful place.

Storybook endings usually are happily ever after, but the real world can be less kind. Psychotherapist and author Belleruth Naparstek once summed it up this way: "Most of us are blandly oblivious to how much comfort we take from our belief that the world is a predictable place, until it demonstrates its random cruelty in some dramatic way."

One of the reasons that your time in the Healing Zone may be emotionally difficult is because of uncertainty about your recovery. While physical recovery can be a bit unpredictable, you may find comfort in knowing that in terms of psychological healing, most people return to their emotional baseline after a time. This process is gradual, however, and not one you can completely control.

I remember the shock of my cancer diagnosis, then a period of intense grieving while I adjusted to my illness and wondered whether my prognosis would turn out to be very grave. After this, my emotions fluctuated. For the most part, they were more blunted than usual—not in the way that shock anesthetizes initially but more subtly. I wasn't depressed, but I certainly didn't feel as happy and optimistic as I usually do. I was in a sort of emotional no-man's-land. It reminded me of a children's nursery rhyme.

When you're up, you're up,
And when you're down, you're down,
But when you're only halfway up,
You're neither up nor down.

This blunting of emotions is normal. It may last for weeks or months as you work to physically and emotionally recover. Healing is a process that sometimes moves forward, sometimes loses ground, and still other times leaves you feeling as though you were stuck somewhere in the middle.

For some people, emotions go off-kilter because of chemical changes in the body after illness or injury or because of side effects from treatment. Cancer treatments, in particular, are notorious for causing emotional upheaval as they alter testosterone and estrogen levels (in both men and women). Pain medications and sleep aids can worsen mood, too.

Cluster symptoms such as fatigue, pain, insomnia, depression, and anxiety may be present to varying degrees in people who are physically healing. These symptoms not only occur together, they also can directly influence each other. For example, someone in pain may not sleep well, which can lead to fatigue. The combination of fatigue and pain can contribute to feelings of

Grief versus Depression

It's important to distinguish between grief and depression. Here's how to tell the difference.

Grief

- Causes sleep disturbances, changes in appetite, reduced ability to concentrate, reduced interest in social activities, and changes in usual behavior patterns (e.g., more irritability or anger)
- Generally waxes and wanes; may vacillate between feelings of hope and sadness; still able to enjoy activities

Depression

- Causes similar symptoms to grief, along with feelings of hopelessness, helplessness, worthlessness, and guilt; in some cases, may trigger thoughts of suicide
- Constant, intense sadness that affects most or all aspects of life; unable to enjoy activities

sadness and even depression. It's a vicious cycle, and recognizing it is the first step to breaking it. Later in this chapter, I will offer specific suggestions about how to deal with emotional issues that may be caused or worsened by the medical world in which you now find yourself.

Dealing with the Day-to-Day

Throughout your journey in the Healing Zone, the real world also will influence your emotions. Daily stress is inevitable, and its sources are many.

I remember a conversation I once had with a neighbor boy who was 11 years old at the time. He said, "I can't wait to be a grown-up because then I won't have so much stress!" When I asked him about the things in his life that were stressful, he listed a host of trials and tribulations, such as not having enough time to play and getting too much homework. While his worries might seem trivial against the backdrop of serious illness, they are a reflection of what all of us go through, regardless of age. Small annoyances and aggravations are a constant presence in our lives.

Along with these daily irritations, we might experience a more significant source of stress. Shortly after I finished chemotherapy and almost immediately after I returned to work part-time, a former physician-colleague began to stalk me. As is true for many victims of stalkers, I still don't exactly know why I became a target. What I surmise is that this man, with whom I'd had a strictly professional relationship, had developed some type of serious psychiatric disorder. When he contacted me after several years of not communicating, we engaged in a short conversation that seemed normal enough. He told me that he was relocating, and he wanted to talk with me about seeking employment in the Boston health community. I agreed to meet with him.

When he came to my office, I sensed almost immediately that something was wrong, though I couldn't discern what it was. Nevertheless, I truthfully told him that there weren't any openings at my hospital that he would qualify for. I ended the meeting quickly and wished him well. Unfortunately, his behavior escalated. He would show up at my workplace unannounced or spend hours sitting across the street at the local Starbucks. He sent strange e-mails and called my home and office. On at least one occasion, the security staff at my hospital escorted him out of the building and gave him a formal written notice that if he were to return, he would be trespassing.

Finally, I called the police. A detective from the Framingham Police Department came to see me. I explained what had happened, that my staff and I felt uncomfortable, and that we didn't know whether this man was capable of violence. Not surprisingly, there wasn't much the detective could do. But he did assure me that he would try to track down this man and strongly urge him to cease contacting me.

As you can imagine, the whole situation was incredibly stressful. Though I wanted to tell the detective that stress wasn't healthy for me as I was trying to heal, I remained silent on that point and just let him do his job. (I doubt he had any idea I'd been ill, though there was one telltale sign—the extremely short hair that follows complete hair loss during chemotherapy.) A few days later, the detective arrived at my office to tell me that he had tracked down my stalker and had strongly discouraged him from bothering me. While the stalking didn't stop right away, I suspect the detective's intervention dampened my former colleague's enthusiasm for contacting me. Eventually, he gave up.

The Positive Side of Negative Emotions

Mood Maxim #3: Negative emotions are an inevitable part of your journey through the Healing Zone. Though an abundance of them can hamper physical recovery, you can use them to your advantage to help focus on Super Healing.

Healing doesn't occur in a vacuum. Real-world stressors, whether minor or major, do have an impact on the healing process. So an important question is, "If I feel stressed, worried, or sad, can I use this to my advantage?

In her book *The Human Side of Cancer: Living with Hope, Coping with Uncertainty,* psychiatrist Jimmie Holland, MD, cautions readers against what she describes as the "tyranny of positive thinking." She writes:

> The present-day tyranny of positive thinking sometimes victimizes people. . . . Trying to get you to "put on a happy face," to pretend you are feeling confident when in fact you are feeling tremendously fearful and upset, can have a downside. By feigning confidence and ease about your illness and its treatment, you may cut off help and support from others. You may also be hiding anxious and depressed feelings that could be alleviated if you told your doctor how you really feel.

In the next section of this chapter, I offer some specific suggestions about how to monitor and improve your mood as you mend. But it's critical to remember that stress breeds more stress. So while paying attention to your emotional state is important, endless worrying about it is not beneficial.

Keep in mind, too, that small "doses" of worry and stress can help sharpen your focus on healing. In *You're Stronger Than You Think*, University of Michigan professor of medicine and psychology Peter Ubel, MD, tells readers:

> When in bad moods . . . people seek out information more thoroughly than when in good moods, and they evaluate arguments more critically. (When bad moods are too extreme, of course, this all breaks down. Severe anxiety and depression are not conducive to clear, focused thinking, nor do they help people deal with negative events.) . . . Many successful athletes say they hate losing more than they love winning. Negative emotions are very good motivators!

In *After Cancer Treatment: Heal Faster, Better, Stronger*, I talk about how frightening a cancer diagnosis is and how we can use those fears as motivation to help us heal. Here's a brief excerpt.

> There is no doubt that cancer is a worrisome diagnosis, regardless of what your prognosis is. We didn't choose cancer, cancer chose us. In her autobiography, English author Margiad Evans wrote, "Our health is a voyage: and every illness is an adventure story." This is one adventure that I would much rather have skipped, but I had no choice. Now all I can do is move forward with my life as a cancer survivor. I don't think that any of us in this ever-growing club, which initiates unwilling members, is completely fearless. I wish that I could take away any fear that you have. I wish that I could eliminate my own fears. But I know I can't. Instead, what I suggest is to use whatever fear you have as a means of motivating yourself to do the best job that you can to heal. If you have to live with demons, make them work for you. Make them part of the healing process.
>
> By far, my greatest inspiration comes from my patients and those individuals I have met through my work who have dealt with tremendous adversity—cancer as well as other serious illnesses and injuries. I have profound admiration for those whom I have watched live through some truly devastating injuries and illnesses and who seemingly handle their health challenges with grace. I have been an earnest student learning from them for many years. One of these individuals is Trisha Meili, a beautiful young woman, who was raped and beaten. Today her outward appearance, soft voice, and ready smile give very little indication of her enormous suffering. However, on April 19, 1989, when she

arrived in the emergency room, she had been brutally beaten. She had multiple fractures, and her body temperature was 85 degrees. She was comatose and had lost so much blood that the doctors gave her little hope of surviving. Yet she did survive this horrific ordeal after a long recovery period. You probably know Trisha as the Central Park Jogger. In her memoir, Trisha wrote, "I built a life until I was 28, was struck down, and so had to build another. Two lives, and I'm proud of both."

Strategies for Emotional Healing

As part of your Super Healing Plan, I suggest starting with one short-term and one long-term goal to improve your mood. Everyone can benefit from setting goals that help to reduce stress and promote healing. On page 161, I offer examples of goals, but you certainly should feel free to create your own, depending on what you think will help you. As you set your goals, you might want to contemplate the following:

1. Stop worrying about worrying. One of the most important things that you can do for yourself is to not fret over having too much stress or experiencing normal fluctuations in your mood. In his book *Worry,* psychiatrist Edward Hallowell, MD, offers these five strategies for reducing worry:

- Never worry alone—talk with someone you trust.
- Get the facts—the toxic part of worry usually is based on misinformation.
- Make a plan—get the right information.
- Take care of yourself—don't spend so much time worrying that you neglect nurturing yourself.
- Let it go—this is easier to do after you have addressed the first four points.

2. Tackle genuine sources of stress by coming up with a plan. In the case of my stalker, I needed to go through formal channels that involved police intervention. Though I couldn't just get rid of this source of stress, it gave me comfort to take the necessary and appropriate steps to change the situation.

3. Actively try to reduce day-to-day stress. This is a good idea for everyone. Here are some strategies that can help keep stress in check.

- Limit or avoid alcohol.
- Eat a well-rounded diet that is low in fat and rich in fruits and vegetables.

- Get proper rest.
- Share your feelings with trusted family members, friends, or clergy.
- Consider joining a support group (for ideas, see Appendix B).
- Exercise regularly.
- Practice meditation or imagery to help with relaxation.
- Commune with nature.
- Pray, if you are comfortable with this.
- Consider trying acupuncture.
- Get a massage or a manicure.
- Educate yourself about your diagnosis and how you can best help yourself.
- Keep a journal.
- Preserve routines that are comforting.
- Surround yourself with feel-good media (e.g., books, CDs, DVDs).
- Continue hobbies that give you pleasure.
- Set limits with family, friends, and co-workers about what you are able to do.
- Avoid self-blame.

4. Consider whether you could benefit from professional support. It's important to recognize when sadness or worry is a more serious problem that requires the attention of a mental health professional. Review the list of signs and symptoms beginning on page 151. If you think that you might have one of these conditions (clinical depression, anxiety, or post-traumatic stress disorder), be sure to see your doctor for appropriate care. Also talk with your doctor if you are experiencing any of the following:

- Difficulty sleeping well
- Unusual or persistent fatigue
- Persistent pain
- Difficulty exercising
- Medication side effects that may be contributing to mood changes (check everything you are taking, even if it is an over-the-counter drug or a supplement)
- Hormonal, nutritional, or another chemical imbalance

Beyond the four steps listed above, you might try these measures to help foster an emotional state that supports optimal healing.

Short- and Long-Term Mood Goals

Below are some examples of mood goals. Keep in mind that other goals in your Super Healing Plan—such as those for therapeutic exercise and for proper rest—will improve your emotional state, too.

Short-Term

- Buy a book or a CD on meditation and practice daily.
- Make an appointment to talk with your doctor about the emotional effects of your illness or injury.
- Start each morning by reading something positive rather than the newspaper.
- Spend time with kids once a week. (Even watching children play in the park can be very uplifting and relaxing.)
- When you exercise, put on music that is fun and uplifting.
- Read a book with a heartening story and a happy ending.

Long-Term

- Meditate twice a day, every day.
- Make a weekly or monthly appointment to pamper yourself at a spa.
- Avoid watching the television news; instead, read a weekly news magazine that highlights the most important current events, so you don't overload your brain with trauma and drama.
- Join a support group.
- Consult with a mental health professional on a regular basis (weekly or monthly).
- Meet regularly with your spiritual advisor.

Ask someone you trust if she thinks you are depressed or overly anxious. Sometimes it's hard for us to judge our own mood. Getting feedback from another source can be extremely helpful. Someone who has known you for a long time can compare how you behave now to what you were like before your illness or injury. If your emotional baseline has changed, you need to recognize and address it.

Aim for 8 hours of uninterrupted sleep each night. Chronic sleep deprivation will work against your emotional health as well as your physical recovery.

Exercise most days of the week. Physical activity triggers the release of chemicals in your body that will make you feel happier and more energetic.

Feed your brain positive messages. While I was going through cancer treatment, I realized how difficult it was for me to read the newspaper or listen to the news. The saying "If it bleeds, it leads" is true. The news media, in particular, are notorious for stirring up our emotions in a very negative manner. I'm not suggesting that you stop paying attention to what's going on around you. But do be selective about the information that you're taking in. How much of it is hopeful, positive, and fun? Too much drama, whether it's fact or fiction, isn't good for anyone. This goes for the books you read, the movies you watch, and even the people you talk to.

Be kind to yourself. By this I mean don't be overly judgmental about your mood. Anyone who is facing serious illness or injury will have their share of bad days. Sometimes the belief that we can completely, or almost completely, control our emotions is so ingrained that we really need to be vigilant about not getting caught up in it. It simply isn't true. What is true is that as you tend to your emotional health, your physical health will improve as well. The two share an impenetrable bond.

Believe in yourself. Research on resilience and happiness has shown that we tend to "catastrophize" how bad something will be and then underestimate how well we can handle it. One of my favorite studies highlighting this tendency is cited in the book *You're Stronger Than You Think*. The study, which dates back to the 1970s, tracked the levels of happiness in three groups of people: lottery winners who had won as much as $1 million within the previous year (the equivalent of tens of millions of dollars today); motor vehicle accident victims who were paralyzed after their injuries; and regular Joes and Josephines from the same neighborhoods as the other two groups. Those in the last group served as controls.

As you may have guessed, the happiest group was the lottery winners, followed by the regular Joes and Josephines and the accident victims. But as Dr. Ubel explains in his book, "To almost everyone's surprise, the happiness of these three groups didn't differ by very much. The fabulously wealthy lottery winners were barely, almost imperceptibly, happier than the regular Joes and Josephines, who in turn weren't all that much happier than the accident victims." This study confirmed what other research has shown: that people tend to be very resilient, even in the face of serious illness or injury.

Mind Your Mood, Mend Your Body

As you may have noticed, some strategies for managing your mood overlap with other components of the Super Healing Plan (e.g., getting proper rest, engaging in therapeutic exercise). This illustrates how the various pieces of the physical recovery puzzle work synergistically. Put all of them together, and you get a complete picture.

This isn't to say that you must do everything perfectly—that every puzzle piece must line up exactly right. What matters most is that you address both the physical and emotional elements of healing so you can recover as completely and as well as possible.

In the next chapter, we'll discuss how love and social connections affect physical healing. The science on this subject is fascinating. Like mind-body interventions and mood, your personal relationships can help cultivate Super Healing.

REMARKABLE RECOVERY

Valerie Daniell

This happened on March 29, 2000. I was 47 years old. I was on vacation, and I wanted to get up early to watch the sun rise. I remember hurling backward off the bed and landing on my head and neck. It was like a backward somersault. My neck broke immediately. It made an incredible sound. I was in excruciating pain, and I couldn't move anything. It didn't dawn on me what had happened.

My friend who was with me immediately called 911. I had a cervical spinal cord injury and underwent emergency surgery. I went to rehab at Baylor. I was in shock at first. I also went through the other stages of grief, denial, and anger. Because I am a licensed mental health counselor, I knew how to process these stages. I remember one period of crying for 2 days straight. But then I realized I had to fight it. I was not going to let it beat me. Emotionally, I turned all of my energy to focus on my recovery.

I had a hard time in rehab because nothing was happening— nothing was moving. My brother came to visit me from Alaska. I was feeling incredibly sorry for myself, and I said to him, "David, if I could just move one finger, that would help me so much." Then I looked down, and my finger moved! I kept moving my finger constantly, and little by little, other parts of my body began to move. This occurred over several weeks. It was like I was frozen, and I started to thaw.

I was a cheerleader in high school and a dancer in college and graduate school. At the time of my injury, I was very active and athletic—skiing, hiking, biking. I tried to visualize myself dancing, and I used that image to help me during my physical therapy sessions.

The doctors kept telling me they didn't think I would ever walk again. I was told I needed to learn how to live in a wheelchair. My parents were elderly, and they didn't know what to do with me, so they put me in a nursing home. I was dropped into this nursing home, and I thought, "This is awful!"

I lost my job, and my boyfriend of 4 years left me a week after I was injured. He said that he didn't want to be with someone in a wheelchair. Throughout my course, I had this vision of being able to walk again and going up to him and kicking him in the butt.

I had a feeling inside that I would walk again. I didn't know why—I just believed it. I found a phenomenal physical therapist to work with, and I begged my father to pay for it. Slowly, I began to take some steps on a gait-assisted treadmill. Then in September, about 6 months after my injury, I was able to walk with crutches.

Ironically, right after I began to walk, I went through a horrible depression. This lasted for about 2 years. By then, I was living by myself. Even though I had close friends, when I was alone, I was really alone. I hit rock bottom; there was nowhere to go except up. It was a good process for me to go through, because I had never really needed to dig deep into my soul. Ultimately, I think my depression was a very positive thing for me. I made myself look for the rainbow after the storm.

My friends called me Humpty Dumpty. They added a line at the end of the rhyme: "All the King's horses and all the King's men couldn't put Humpty together again. She had to do it herself you see, with the help of friends and family."

A miracle happened to me in 2003—I reconnected with my high school sweetheart. I never thought that a man would be interested in me again. I had this broken body, but my spirit was still strong. He just jumped right into my life like I never expected. His love gave me a whole new perspective on my life.

I had to learn the difference between adjusting to my disability and accepting it. Accepting it took me many years. Once I did accept that I'd probably always have to use crutches to walk, I was able to really get back into life. It took me too long to get there, but I'm there now. Today my motto is "attitude is everything."

Chapter 11

Surround Yourself with Loving People

I encourage my patients who are physically recovering from an illness or injury to set a "love goal" for themselves. It often comes as a surprise to them that a relatively conservative rehabilitation doctor like me would broach this delicate subject, much less recommend something that seems so far afield from what might help with physical recovery. On the surface, giving and receiving love has little in common with Super Healing. Nevertheless, the former is vital to the latter.

I mention this goal when I talk with patients about physical recovery, because a growing body of scientific evidence recognizes love as a potent medicine that can not only prevent illness before it strikes but also help those who are sick heal more quickly and completely. In fact, love can positively affect the quality of your life as well as the quantity of your days.

The research on this is so compelling that renowned heart specialist Dean Ornish, MD, wrote an entire book on the healing power of love and intimacy. In this fascinating bestseller—aptly titled *Love and Survival*—Dr. Ornish observes, "If a new drug had the same impact, virtually every doctor in the country would be recommending it for their patients. It would be malpractice not to prescribe it."

Love Is Good Medicine

When 5-year-old David Eustace started kindergarten, he was thrilled about his new school, his teacher, and his friends. All that would change, quickly and dramatically, when an elderly gentleman who was picking up his grand-child at school accidentally stepped on the gas rather than the brake. His car lurched over the curb onto the sidewalk and directly into a group of children. Eleven people were injured, three from the same family—David, his 3-year-old sister, and his cousin. "I remember after the car hit me," David says. "There was blood all over the wall, and the car just sort of fell into pieces. They put me on a stretcher. I went in an ambulance. Then I went in a helicopter."

Understandably, David's father and mother were devastated. For months, they stayed by their son's side every day and every night at the hospital where he was a patient. They did what loving, caring parents do— they nurtured David and showered him with affection and attention. This helped him to heal. (You'll find David's Remarkable Recovery story at the end of this chapter.)

It makes sense that a child would heal better with devoted parents who are constantly present. But what about adults? How does love affect us?

Neil Sullivan was a 34-year-old firefighter when he became trapped between two fire trucks. Like David, Neil lost one of his legs. He spent weeks in the hospital following his injury. As he recalls, one of the most meaningful experiences of his recovery occurred one evening as he lay in his hospital bed contemplating his fate. Three New York City firemen walked into his room. They had read about Neil in the newspaper. Neil says, "They came just to tell me that they were behind me, thinking of me, and that they wanted to thank me because they had heard that I had gone to the funerals [of their fellow firefighters] after 9/11." Neil is convinced that the love of his family, friends, and colleagues helped him to heal.

Both David and Neil experienced firsthand the healing power of loving, nurturing personal relationships. Scientific studies offer convincing proof that married couples, in particular, tend to be healthier and live longer. Yet even though a loving, monogamous marital partnership can have a positive impact on physical health, many other kinds of human connections are important as well.

For instance, in a study tracking survival rates among Australians, researchers found the strongest survival benefit among those people with several friends and confidants. The reasons for this are not well understood but may have something to do with the fact that peer relationships encourage healthier lifestyles, such as staying physically active, not smoking, avoiding excessive alcohol consumption, and so on. Another reason may be that people who are able to form lasting friendships have greater "social capital." Friendships are just one component of social capital, which is defined as "connections among individuals." A society of people who are talented and industrious but relatively isolated is poor in social capital.

Though social capital isn't always positive (as in the case of gangs and white supremacy groups), it usually is beneficial for health and survival.

Connections to friends, loved ones, the community, and the environment may bring about physical changes that improve health and promote healing. Some scientists hypothesize that levels of oxytocin, a hormone produced by the hypothalamus in the brain, increase during positive social interactions. Oxytocin may be best known for helping mothers and babies bond during breastfeeding. Oxytocin's role in other relationships is not as well understood, but higher levels during positive social engagements may result in health benefits. Other hormones and biological compounds in our bodies may reinforce the link between affection and wellness.

Back in Chapter 2, I referred to an article by Lewis Mehl-Madrona, MD, titled "Connectivity and Healing: Some Hypotheses about the Phenomenon and How to Study It." Dr. Mehl-Madrona explores how connection makes a difference in healing—in part because of the concept of "coherence," which is the coming together (in a unified manner) of many different healing influences.

Psychiatrist Edward Hallowell, MD, believes that connection among humans has such a significant impact on health that he wrote a fascinating book on the topic, appropriately titled *Connect*. In it he states, "Connection is an essential vitamin. You can't live without it."

While some critics maintain that human biology—including health and healing—is not influenced by human bonds, the scientific evidence strongly suggests otherwise. One rather clever study that appeared in the *Journal of the American Medical Association* examined whether social ties would affect susceptibility to the common cold. For this study, researchers placed drops of two different viruses into the noses of healthy volunteers. Taking into account a variety of demographic factors—including age, gender, weight, and so on—the researchers still concluded that people with more social ties were much less likely to become sick.

How Relationships Affect Physical Healing

Since this is a book about physical healing, you may be wondering what the scientific literature has to say about whether and how love and connection support the healing process. Perhaps just as interestingly, what happens to physical recovery when you're surrounded by people who aren't especially nurturing and supportive? Could the toxic people in your life—and most of us have them—actually keep you from healing optimally?

In a remarkable study on this very topic, published in the *Archives of General Psychiatry,* researchers evaluated wound healing among couples.

Each participating pair was admitted two times to a hospital research unit. During each admission, the participants were "wounded" with a skin-blistering technique. The researchers recorded how fast the wounds healed and how well the participants produced levels of healing compounds known as cytokines. The couples' relationships were evaluated and rated by the researchers as either "high hostile" or "low hostile."

During the first admission, the couples were encouraged to have a positive interaction with each other. During the second admission, they were given a conflict resolution task that produced a more negative interaction. Not surprisingly, the wounds of the high-hostile couples healed much more slowly, at just 60 percent of the rate among the low-hostile couples. Comparing the two hospital admissions, both groups showed slower rates of healing during the second admission, when stress was higher because of the focus on the conflict-resolution task. Still, the low-hostile couples healed faster.

Based on the results of many studies exploring personal relationships and physical healing and relationships, we know that love and support help recovery and discord hinders it. As the authors of the above study noted:

> Marriage is the central relationship for the majority of adults, and morbidity and mortality are reliably lower for married individuals than unmarried individuals across such diverse health threats as cancer, heart attack, and surgery . . . the simple presence of a spouse is not necessarily protective; a troubled marriage is itself a prime source of stress, while simultaneously limiting the partner's ability to seek support in other relationships.

How Illness Affects Relationships

There is no doubt that illness has an effect on personal relationships. For some, the effect may be very positive. There are many stories of families reuniting after a loved one becomes ill. One woman told me that her bout with ovarian cancer was the clichéd "blessing in disguise" because it brought her estranged adult daughter back into the family fold.

While some relationships will easily endure and even strengthen during a medical crisis, others may suffer. In her book *Finding The Way Home,* author Gayle Heiss writes, "One of the most painful aspects of illness is that, along the way, it can and often does leave people feeling broken, lost, separate—alienated from others and from life as they knew it."

Those of us who have experienced health problems are well aware of their far-reaching consequences. Friends and loved ones cannot and do not embrace the challenge in every instance. Claudia Osborn, the physician who had a cycling accident and sustained a traumatic head injury, addresses this in her memoir by sharing the thoughts of her treasured friend and roommate. As her friend says:

> I blame the injury, not Claudia, for the shell of a person who awoke after two weeks of round-the-clock sleeping. In the acute stages of illness, it's easy to be a good friend—exhausting but rewarding to nurse a loved one back to health. But her health never returned, and chronic care takes tenacious strength when you're also battling grief. I often feel unequal to the challenge. . . . I will support her efforts to improve and be here when she comes home, but I cannot endlessly play the selfless, devoted friend. I do not believe the emotional truth of those who watch their relationship change from that of equals to one of parent-child without protest, sorrow, and rage.

Karen Horowitz is a patient of mine and a three-time breast cancer survivor. After her first diagnosis, her best friend of 25 years struggled to cope with the situation and ended up calling less often. By Karen's third diagnosis, her best friend was ignoring her completely, and their decades-long friendship collapsed. Another friend who couldn't face her illness was more straightforward. She told her, "I can't handle this and I won't be calling you, but I'll check in with our mutual friends to see how you are doing." Karen respected this woman's candor, and though the two didn't keep in touch during the time that she was in the Healing Zone, they have remained friends.

In contrast to these two women, Karen's husband was a rock. He encouraged her all along the way, helping her to become a breast cancer advocate who now travels throughout the United States and was recently chosen as an ambassador for the American Cancer Society. Karen credits her husband's—and her daughters'—unwavering support with helping her to heal through three cancer diagnoses and form many new friendships with people whom she has met through her advocacy work.

For Karen, her husband's support extended to their physical relationship, in which he remained loving and nonjudgmental about the changes to her body—including a mastectomy with breast reconstruction. But for many couples, illness or injury can have a major impact on physical intimacy, for both physical and emotional reasons. For example, sexual desire and performance can suffer because of either the underlying condition or the treatments. (Some cancer treatments can induce early menopause in women, while for men, problems with having erections is a common medication side effect.) Pain and fatigue are common during physical recovery, and both symptoms can interfere with intimacy.

Physical changes can have psychological effects as well. Scars, amputations, and weight loss or gain may leave an ill partner feeling less desirable—or a well partner less desiring. Other potential emotional issues can arise from a shift in the balance of power in a relationship as one partner takes on more of a caregiving role.

Chris Penrod was a 29-year-old mechanic when he suffered serious burns in a fire at work. He says that taking off his shirt in front of a woman is hard because he has tremendous scars on his body. "When I was in the hospital, I had a girlfriend, and she left," Chris explains. "So dating again . . . involved whether women were going to leave because of how I look." It hasn't been easy for Chris, but as he says, "I have a girlfriend now who doesn't mind it. Like she says, we all have our problems." (You can read more of Chris's Remarkable Recovery story on page 224.)

One of my patients is a young woman who underwent breast cancer treatment several years ago. She has an excellent prognosis and is doing well in all aspects of her life, with the exception of resuming an intimate relationship with her husband. She tells me that she is uncomfortable with physical intimacy because she no longer feels attractive. Her surgery left a small scar on her breast, while chemotherapy caused her to lose her hair and gain weight. Though her hair has grown back, she remains self-conscious about the scar and the weight gain. She makes no overtures to her husband because she doesn't want to "lead him on."

Suzy Becker is another woman who struggled with physical intimacy following brain surgery. She wrote about how it affected her relationship and how her partner, Karen, "needed to make love to feel loved" while she needed to "feel loved to make love." Becker describes this as the "lovers' catch-22."

Yet many other couples maintain loving, physically intimate relationships despite one partner's illness or injury. Geralyn Lucas wrote about how she and her husband had sex almost immediately following her mastectomy for breast cancer. Though Geralyn wasn't sure how her husband would react sexually, he led the way, and she reciprocated. Geralyn describes the experience and how it helped her realize the depth of her husband's love for her.

> I put on some perfume. And I line my lips with lipstick. I can't even feel Tyler's hand when he puts it on the bright red diagonal scar across my chest. In fact, I have been walking into strangers with my reconstructed right boob because I cannot feel where it starts.

But the great thing about sex is that it's like riding a bicycle. I know that Tyler still loves me—my laugh, our conversations—but will he still be turned on?

Yes, yes, and definitely yes. I cannot believe that Tyler wants me so much.

The way he is kissing me and touching me, I know that it's not my hair or my boob that ever made him fall in love with me. It was my mojo. It was always there, just waiting for me to meet it.

After Tyler and I have sex again I feel so hot that I still can't get that Shania Twain song out of my head: *Man, I feel like a woman!*

Geralyn and I met when both of us were on NBC doing a televised segment on breast cancer. When I told her that I was going to use her story in a chapter on love for my own book, she laughed and said that it was all true.

Giving and Receiving Love

It is not entirely clear whether it is better to give love or to receive love. Though the latter might seem more beneficial, research offers compelling evidence in favor of the former. For example, in a study involving nursing home residents, those who took care of the plants in their rooms lived 5 to 7 years longer than those who had plants but weren't responsible for them. In a separate study involving older couples, which appeared in the journal *Psychological Science,* individuals who gave support to others were more likely to live longer.

Relationships, of course, require the participation of two people, which intrinsically fosters a natural giving and receiving of affection and practical support. Usually, the greater the commitment of one partner to the nurturing of the other, the stronger the union. In many relationships, though, one person does most of the nurturing. This is not always problematic or unnatural, such as in the case of a parent-child bond. But in liaisons in which both partners should be equal in their affection for and support of each other, sometimes one person does more of the giving.

Relationships do have an ebb and flow to them, in which the amount of nurturing needed and provided depends on many factors. Serious illness or injury certainly can bring about changes in how someone gives and receives love. During my treatment for cancer, I experienced an outpouring of love from my friends and colleagues. Perfect for healing, right? Well, yes and no. I very much appreciated their devotion and kindness, but sometimes it was hard to accept. For instance, I had always been in charge of cooking my children's meals. When I was ill, friends cooked for us. I was grateful for their assistance, while at the same time, I wanted to be the one who tended to my children's needs.

I am not the only one who has found it more difficult to give than to receive. Couples therapists Harville Hendrix, PhD, and Helen LaKelly Hunt, PhD, address this issue in their book *Receiving Love*.

> The common wisdom is that romantic relationships would stay happy if people did a better job of giving to each other. But that's not what we've discovered. We've found that many people need to do a better job of receiving the gifts their partners are already offering. It's surprising how often the compliments, appreciations, and encouragements of well-intentioned partners make no dent in the armor of an unhappy partner. The compliments are brushed off, the votes of confidence are discounted, and the words of encouragement fall on deaf ears.

Drs. Hendrix and Hunt—who are married to each other—go on to say:

> Since connection depends upon a desire and willingness both to give yourself and to receive the other, not receiving in a relationship is like jamming a stick into the spoke of a bicycle wheel—it stops the action.

Some couples maintain a comfortable balance between giving and receiving only to find that the balance shifts when one partner enters the Healing Zone. This can wreak havoc on their relationships.

Two cornerstones of serious illness, dependency and suffering, can shake the foundation of even the strongest personal bond. But as psychologist Harriet Lerner, PhD, reminds us, they are a necessary and important aspect of the human condition. In her book *The Dance of Connection,* Dr. Lerner writes, "Sooner or later harsh experience teaches us how much we need each other. The only aspect of either that's really shameful is the persistent and false societal belief that people can bootstrap their way to health, wealth, and happiness."

Nevertheless, a serious medical condition can and often does marginalize a person's role in a relationship. A parent may become less essential to her children as they begin to rely on others. Or an adolescent may become increasingly reliant on a parent, thus challenging the normal transition into adulthood.

Back in high school, a good friend of mine shared with me how upset he was that after breaking both of his arms in a car accident, he needed to rely on his mother to help him go to the bathroom. As high-school kids sometimes do, he described this in graphic detail. Even as a teenager, I understood that he was making the transition to manhood, and having his mother be responsible for wiping his bottom—much as she did when he was a baby—was extremely difficult for him.

All relationships are subject to change, though perhaps only temporarily, when one partner is in the Healing Zone. The challenge is to be able to graciously accept the love and nurturing of others while at the same time continuing to try to nurture them in return.

When People Aren't Paying Attention, Don't Assume They Don't Care

Some kinds of medical crises seem to instantly bring people together. When someone is seriously injured in a car accident or diagnosed with cancer, for example, loved ones rally to provide emotional and practical support. But many other serious medical conditions don't elicit the same level of empathy and aid. This subdued response from family members and friends almost always is the result of a lack of understanding about the diagnosis and symptoms, as well as the nature of a person's needs.

For instance, a young woman with multiple sclerosis may appear healthy to those around her, even though she's struggling physically because of muscle weakness. Walking can be difficult, as can carrying out daily activities such as taking care of her home or climbing the stairs to her office. Though she wishes for others to be more attentive and helpful, her family and friends view her as self-sufficient and not needing either emotional or practical support.

Even with a crisis diagnosis such as cancer, loved ones may provide support up to a certain point and then withdraw once they perceive that the crisis has passed. With cancer in particular, this retreat often begins when the patient is at his lowest point physically—at the end of chemotherapy or other treatment.

Anyone who's in the Healing Zone can benefit from emotional and possibly practical support. Even if you're able to function completely independently, without relying on others, now might be a good time to accept help so you can invest your energy in recovering as well as possible. For instance, if you are able to do your grocery shopping but it leaves you too tired for exercise, it isn't a good trade-off. Exercise is much more important than grocery shopping to someone in the Healing Zone. Tasks that wear you out rather than help you heal should be delegated whenever possible.

Sometimes it may feel like an energy drain to engage friends because you find yourself repeating the same information over and over. It gets tiresome. But my colleague Paula Rauch, MD, a psychiatrist at Harvard Medical School, has a terrific solution to this dilemma. She suggests designating a loved one as your "minister of information," who will share with others how you are doing and what you need. Through her, you can stay in touch with your social circle without the emotional drain of telling your story again and again. Your minister of information should talk with only those people whom you select or approve of and provide only the details you want others to know. This person also can assist with your love goals by planning outings with friends and other events. Your minister of information helps you stay connected without making you do all of the work yourself. She wants to help, so let her.

As you consider your love goals, decide who would be a good minister of information for you. This person should be trustworthy, organized, and kind. More than likely, the person you choose will be honored and will have been trying to figure out ways to support you.

Recruiting a minister of information is not meant to be a barrier to keep you from reaching out to others. Rather, this person is a facilitator. You still want to personally engage family members and friends as much as you're able; often, this is as simple as telling them more about what you currently are going through.

Confiding in people you trust frequently leads to inquiries about how they might help. If they ask, give them specific answers so their assistance truly is useful. If they don't offer, you might ask them outright. Most people truly enjoy helping others, as you probably do. While asking for support is taking a bit of a risk, keep in mind that the person you're asking might not have offered for fear of being rebuffed. Though some people might not jump at the chance to help, most people who are not forthcoming simply are waiting for you to take the initiative and tell them how they can best nurture you during this time.

Passengers to Join You on Your Healing Journey

As you build your social capital, consider which of your personal connections are most nurturing and which are potentially toxic. On your journey through the Healing Zone, you want the most caring and supportive passengers to accompany you. If you have a close relationship that is not going well, you might want to consider separating yourself from that person—for the time being, at least—and not inviting him or her on your journey.

Of course, this might not be desirable or feasible if the person with whom you are in conflict is your partner or a family member. In such cases, honest and straightforward communication about the state of your relationship and the need to make adjustments might be the best solution. In her book *Saying What's Real,* self-described relationship coach Susan Campbell endorses this direct approach.

> In relationships, as in life, change is the only constant. So why do we have so much difficulty embracing the need for moment-to-moment course correction in relating with others? I think the answer has something to do with our outdated notions about change. Most of us still see stability as the norm and change as a problem. We like things to be predictable—"no surprises." In reality, people's feelings and wants change constantly. As long as we resist this fact, we will not learn the very important lesson of how to allow for constant change within an ongoing relationship. The ability to embrace change in the context of long-term stability is one of the biggest relationship challenges of our time. "Can we talk. . . ?" will help you develop this important skill.

In some relationships, only one person is willing to try to make changes. Good communication may not be possible or effective.

In her book *How One of You Can Bring the Two of You Together,* relationship expert Susan Page says that the most important component of a successful relationship is not an absence of challenges but an abundance of goodwill. Page writes, "Couples who thrive exhibit a fundamental goodwill toward each other. They want the best for each other. Even in conflicts, they don't feel like adversaries but like allies, striving to maintain trust and safety within the bounds of their twosome."

Page goes on to observe that "goodwill begets goodwill, but someone has to start." Her advice: "If you can 'act as if' you love and adore your spouse and you are happy in your relationship, even if only for 5 minutes a day or 2 hours a week, you may be doing more to 'solve your problems' than if you spent 5 hours 'working things out' . . . If you start to behave as you would if you were happy, and make your body behave as you would if you were happy, your feelings will actually follow suit."

When the Journey Involves Children

As you travel through the Healing Zone, you may encounter some passengers who are reluctant to join you. Illness is a family affair, and not everyone will ride without complaint. Children especially may be reticent and perhaps worried. As news correspondent Betty Rollin once wrote, "Disease may score a direct hit on only one member of a family, but shrapnel tears the flesh of the others."

My colleague Dr. Rauch founded and directs a program at Massachusetts General Hospital called PACT (Parenting at a Challenging Time). She also is the co-author of *Raising an Emotionally Healthy Child When a Parent Is Sick*. When I asked her what she most wants parents to know about how to help their children, she offered the following:

> I encourage parents to focus on three areas of a child's life: the child's schedule, family time, and communication. Have a pre-dictable daily and weekly routine, because this makes the world feel safer to a child. Turn off the phone during meals, and protect family time from too many visitors or phone conversations about a parent's health status. Be honest and simple about illness expla-nations, and encourage children to ask their own questions. Welcome all questions warmly, and try to tease out the real question a child has before launching into an answer that may not address the real concern or confusion. When you focus on these three areas, often the parent's illness recedes into the background, and the focus turns to the child's healthy development.

In her book, Dr. Rauch advises parents to appoint not only a minister of information but also a "captain of kindness." These two people can work together to support your family. The minister of information directs people who want to help to the captain of kindness, whose job is to orga-nize the well-wishers. This service can be extremely useful for you and your family.

For example, when a friend asks, "What can I do to help?" you may feel awkward saying that you need someone to take your children to soccer practice or a movie. Your captain of kindness can act as a buffer and steer people in the right direction so your freezer doesn't fill up with too many casseroles. Even if you don't have young children, choosing a minister and a captain can free you to focus on healing. Take time now to call two friends who would be delighted to claim these roles. It's a great way to make contact with them and foster physical healing through the power of love and connection.

In her book *When a Parent Has Cancer,* Wendy Schlessel Harpham, MD—who was diagnosed with non-Hodgkins lymphoma as a young mother—reminds us that "the greatest gift you can give your children is not protection from change, loss, pain, or stress, but the confidence and tools to cope and grow with all that life has to offer them." If you have children, the following strategies might help make them more comfortable, confident passengers on your journey through the Healing Zone.

Tell them the truth, including the real name of your condition. All children have a good sense of when someone is being honest with them. Always tell them the truth. Don't keep your diagnosis a secret. You don't need to tell them everything at once, as they may not have the attention span to absorb all of the details, but what you do share should be factual. Remember, you are your child's best source of information. As Dr. Harpham notes, "When the facts are couched in love and hopefulness, you can guide your children toward a life-enhancing perception of reality. In the end, that's what parenting is all about."

Stick with their routines as much as possible. If you are in the process of raising your children, you have every right to be worried about them and their future. In her book *After Breast Cancer,* Hester Hill Schnipper—an oncology social worker and breast cancer survivor—offers this reassurance.

> It is very likely that your children will have adjusted quickly and managed reasonably well during your months of treatment. I and colleagues in my hospital's Department of Psychiatry worked on a longitudinal study of the reactions of children to a mother's breast cancer, and we have found, over and over, that children who are given age-appropriate information and whose routines remain consistent do very well. Indeed, their mothers say that it sometimes seems as if the children actually forget about the cancer and so are startled when they catch a glimpse of a bald head or are told of a doctor's appointment. They do not really forget, of course, nor are they in denial. It is simply that their healthy defenses are working well, protecting them as they go about their daily business of growing up.

Participate when you can, and explain when you can't. Children need to know what to expect from parents and other adults in their lives. So tell your children what you can and can't do, especially as it pertains to family routines and special occasions. Let them know that your love and devotion are unchanged despite spending time going to the doctor or attending to other aspects of your illness. Explain who will be there to help them. Remind them that you still are their parent, despite your condition.

Remember that your children will follow your emotional lead. Research shows that children take their cues from their parents—which means that in all likelihood, your children will do as well as you do. If you are positive, hopeful, honest, and communicative, your children likely will react in a similar fashion. Listen to them. Stay in tune with what is happening at home and at school. Seek professional care if your child's problems are beyond the scope of what is normal and what you are able to address.

On the other hand, don't be surprised if your children cope even better than you anticipated. I remember one occasion when I received a card from the mother of one of my daughter's classmates. In it she wrote, "I thought it was so brave of your daughter to share such personal and difficult news about your illness with her classmates." I was surprised, though not at all upset, that my daughter had announced my illness publicly. I had explained to my children that some people—especially their friends and classmates—might mention that they knew people who had died of cancer. I didn't want this to scare them, so I told them to be ready for such comments and to say that my doctors thought they could help me. Sure enough, my daughter's proclamation prompted other children to chime in with tales of relatives who had lost their cancer battles.

You can't predict every situation that your child will encounter, but being as candid and as optimistic as possible can make all the difference in helping them to deal with what is happening to you.

You Are Not a Burden to Your Loved Ones

Perhaps you feel as though you're relying too heavily on family and friends or even "using" them on your journey through the Healing Zone. Using people suggests that someone is being disingenuous and perhaps even dishonest. This most definitely is not the case. Surrounding yourself with loved ones who nurture and support you, and whom you in turn nurture and support, is integral not only to healing well but also to leading a worthwhile life. Just as they are helping you recover, you are helping them by graciously receiving their affection and support.

Family members and friends are not the only connections that can make a difference while you're in the Healing Zone. Dr. Hallowell identifies the following "12 points of connection":

1. Family of origin

2. Immediate family

3. Friends and community

4. Work, mission, activity

5. Beauty (e.g., music, art, literature)

6. The past (knowing where you came from and how you connect to your descendants through religion, ethnicity, and so on)

7. Nature and special places

8. Pets and other animals

9. Ideas and information (e.g., thinking about ideas, discussing them with others, connecting with them)

10. Institutions and organizations

11. Whatever is beyond knowledge (e.g., spirituality)

12. Yourself (create a healing, loving, nonjudgmental dialogue in your own mind about yourself)

As you read through the above list, think of the ways in which you can strengthen the connections in your own life. Even if you don't adopt the following suggestions as formal goals, try making them a part of your life in order to nurture yourself and your loved ones.

Take time to greet people you meet, even if they are strangers. Start by saying something pleasant and seeing how they respond. You likely will get at least a smile; if you do, take advantage of it and open a conversation. Find out people's names and something about their lives. The next time you see them, you'll have a connection based on your reaching out to them in the past.

Make spending time with family and friends a priority. Your journey through the Healing Zone likely has taken a lot of time and energy. Perhaps you've lost touch with certain people who are meaningful in your life. Reach out to them. They probably miss you as much as you miss them.

Plan a date with yourself, with the objective of simply showering love on yourself. Treat yourself to whatever will make you feel special and nurtured. You could go to a play or concert, have a picnic in the park, or get pampered at a spa. This is your time, so plan it just the way you want it to go. Feel free to invite someone else if you'd like company.

Defining Love Goals

I suggest creating at least two love goals, one short-term and one long-term, to help facilitate the healing process. But before you do, let's consider the points of connection and how they apply to you.

The idea behind a love goal is to increase your social capital while at the same time avoiding additional stress. Someone who is shy by nature might be anxious about joining a community group that's all strangers. Likewise, someone who is having trouble with mobility may be reluctant to go to a park and commune with nature. Your love goals should be comfortable and reasonable for you to accomplish. (See page 180 for several examples of goals.)

There is no doubt that making new connections can be challenging

Short- and Long-Term Love Goals

Compared with the rest of your goals, your love goals will be intensely personal. Review the following examples, then consider how you might formulate goals to build and strengthen your connections with those around you.

Remember that as you follow the Super Healing Plan, you will create one short-term love goal to start, then update this goal monthly. So over the next year, you will complete 12 short-term goals. You also will have two long-term goals for the year, one for every 6 months.

Short-Term

- Reestablish contact with five old friends.

- Write a love letter to your partner and each of your children.

- Join a support group and attend the meetings.

- Plan a weekly date with a friend (it needn't be the same person every week).

- Meet a friend for a walk at least once a week.

- Warmly greet the "angels" in your life. Take time to learn their names and a bit about them.

- Sign up for a class (e.g., yoga, woodworking, journal writing).

- Attend at least two events in your community (e.g., pancake breakfast, school concert, town meeting, bingo).

- Sign up to participate in an event that supports a charitable cause (e.g., walkathon, crafts fair).

while you are in the Healing Zone. In her memoir, Joni Rodgers—a young woman diagnosed with non-Hodgkin's lymphoma—recited a pretend conversation that she might have with a new acquaintance: "Hi, I'm Joni, and I'm a sucking black hole of emotional need right now. My hobbies are taking drugs, napping, and calling people I hardly know for emergency child care. Wanna be my friend?"

I like this conversation because it's clever and also because it so accurately reflects how I felt while I was in the Healing Zone. Normally I am an

- Volunteer in your community (e.g., school library, local hospital, senior center) one morning or afternoon a week.

Long-Term

- Resume intimacy with your partner at a level that is satisfying for both of you.

- Maintain weekly contact with three old friends.

- Continue attending support group meetings.

- Plan and take a vacation with family or friends to a place you have never been.

- Exercise with a partner at least once a week.

- Continue taking a class or sign up for another one in which you learn something new.

- Join a group in your community (e.g., Rotary International, Junior League, Girl Scouts).

- Volunteer to help organize (not just participate in) an upcoming charitable event.

- Sign up for a sports team or attend "open gym" at least once a week.

- Join or become more active in a spiritual institution (e.g., church, synagogue, mosque).

outgoing person who likes to meet new people. But when I was ill, I felt vulnerable and was much less open to connecting with others, especially if I didn't know them very well.

For your love goals, you could focus on making new connections. But if you're feeling vulnerable, as I did, you might want to work on the connections you already have. This could mean calling an old friend with whom you've lost touch or writing a loving letter to your partner or one of your children.

Most of us have many people in our lives with whom we could connect, only we are too busy or too distracted to do so. Maureen Pratt, who has lived with lupus for more than a decade, writes about these vital connections in *Peace in the Storm.*

> The postal carrier who delivers your mail. The trash collector who gathers your garbage. The nurse who draws your blood. The friend who brings you supper when you're too sick to cook for yourself. The doctor who squeezes you into his already packed schedule. The stranger who opens a door for you . . .
>
> Each day, in great ways and small, we are surrounded by angels. Not the celestial creatures with halos and wings, but the flesh and blood angels who help us and give us encouragement, even if we don't know their names.

Pausing for even a few minutes to chat with the people with whom you come into contact over the course of a day can help you feel much more connected to them and to the world around you. These brief interactions may lead to deeper bonds over time, as you learn the names and the life stories of these "flesh and blood angels."

As you work to increase or strengthen your connections, avoid overrelying on the Internet. Often it's thought of as the ultimate connection source because of its speed and far-reaching capacity. Actually, though, the Internet can decrease your social capital. For a study published in the journal *American Psychologist,* researchers tracked the effects of the Internet on more than 150 people during their first 1 to 2 years online. Overall, the study participants used the Internet quite extensively for communication. "Nonetheless," the scientists wrote, "greater use of the Internet was associated with declines in participants' communication with family members in the household, declines in the size of their social circle, and increases in their depression and loneliness."

Connect and Conquer

Social capital, love, and all of the connections that surround you can facilitate your efforts to Super Heal. As physician and poet Oliver Wendell Holmes once said, "The sound of a kiss is not so loud as that of a cannon, but its echo lasts a great deal longer."

Of course, serious illness or injury can complicate relationships or cause feelings of loneliness and isolation. Consciously and deliberately counteracting this tendency can make your passage through the Healing Zone much smoother and quicker. Dr. Hallowell sums up this point quite nicely in his book *Connect*: "Life is loss . . . To oppose the pain of loss, we use a human glue, the force of love. The force of love creates our many different connections. This is what saves us all."

REMARKABLE RECOVERIES

David Eustace

David was attending his first week of kindergarten when he was struck by a car outside his school. His father, Paul, describes what happened.

On October 1, 2004, David was coming out of his kindergarten when an elderly man lost control of his car and came up on the sidewalk. He struck David and 11 other people, including my daughter and my niece.

The second I got a call from my wife's cell phone and someone else was on the other end, I knew there was something seriously wrong. The officer on the other end told me that there was an accident, and it was just like your worst fear comes true. By this time, I was kind of losing it. I was at work, and I just bolted to my car and headed right to the hospital. I beat the helicopter and the ambulances there.

David finally came in. My daughter, Nicole, and my niece, Elizabeth, came in, too. Nicole was alert and awake and talking. She was screaming, crying.

The emergency room intern came over to me and said to me, "You should go see your son. He might not make it." And when he told me this, it didn't register. He came over and told me again, and this time it was like a pain. I went over and I saw David, and I asked him, "Are you all right, buddy?" He just looked at me and said, "No." It was the first time he'd ever said no when I asked him if he was all right.

Nicole and Elizabeth were in the hospital for a couple of days. Elizabeth broke her leg. Nicole had a fractured eye socket. David, on the other hand, lost his left leg above the knee, and his right leg was nearly severed.

David was in the ICU for 3 weeks. He was in and out of consciousness, and he was delusional for about 3 days. Then he started coming out of it, and it was up to my wife and me who was going to tell him that he didn't have his leg anymore.

I finally told him one night. He had a feeling; I know he had a feeling that it was gone. We kind of hid it from him, but I think he just knew. At first he said, "I don't want a leg with no foot." He said that for about 2 weeks. And then it was incredible. One day he basically said that he had accepted it. He said something like, "I can live with this. This isn't so bad." And there was just a sigh of relief when he said it. It was like the first hint that maybe he was going to be all right.

We spent 3 months at Massachusetts General Hospital. The first week I was a mess. My wife wasn't. She was solid through the whole thing. For about the first week I had some sort of amnesia. I don't remember a lot, and it wasn't due to alcohol or drugs or anything. It was just some sort of strain. I didn't go to sleep for 3 days after the accident, so that might have had something to do with it.

David was finally discharged from the ICU, and we went up to the 17th floor of Mass General for the next 2½ months. And, you know, we were asking all kinds of questions about prostheses and stuff like that, and he finally started coming back to himself. I mean, he had a lot of pain, and he was on morphine. He wasn't eating, and he was vomiting all the time. But finally, he came through it, and he got out of the hospital in January.

There was still a question about the other leg, whether they would be able to save it. It wasn't until 8 months afterward, after the doctor installed a plate in his leg, that we found out that the leg was going to be saved.

David went back to school in a wheelchair, and he wasn't self-conscious. He'd scoot around, using his hands to push himself along on his bum in the classroom. Then I made a chair for him so that he could be moved from one station to another in his classroom. He played T-ball in his wheelchair, and he was hitting better than a lot of the other kids who weren't in wheelchairs. Every time, the first swing he'd hit the ball.

Eventually he got his prosthesis. He mastered it within 2 weeks, and he was walking. They told us that he might never be able to figure out how to run with it, because a lot of above-the-knee amputees never figure out how to run. But I remember coming home about 2 months after he got the prosthesis, and my wife said, "Look at this," and he was running.

The most important thing is that he did not lose who he was. He's still the same kid. He's still the exact same kid as he was before this happened. He has numerous good friends, about three or four really close friends. He's playing T-ball. He's running. He's going to start playing basketball. He can't skate, he can't ride a bike, he can't keep up with the other kids a lot of times, but he doesn't complain about it and he doesn't get upset. He was always a special kid.

REMARKABLE RECOVERIES

Neil Sullivan

Neil Sullivan was a 34-year old fireman following in his father's foot-steps on a fateful night in the summer of 2005. Here's his story, in his own words.

It was a Saturday night, and the bell hit at about 1 o'clock in the morning. There are certain times you have a feeling of what you're going to. This night, with the way the phone calls were coming in, people saying they were seeing heavy fire blowing out of the windows of the house, we were pretty confident that there was going to be a fire going on when we got there.

The company that I was on was one of the first to pull up at the house. As we were getting our gear together and going up the front steps, the family was running out and screaming because some family members were still in bed sleeping. Our initial attack was to get all the people out of the house. Once we did that, we started running our hose lines into the house.

At this point, the captain who was in charge started to call in for neighboring communities to come and help us, because it was a good-size Victorian house and he knew that we had a lot of work ahead of us. The crew that I was with took the hose line into the kitchen, where there was some heavy fire.

Usually your tank gives you somewhere between 20 and 30 minutes of air, so there was a point that my alarm was going off, telling me that I probably had 5 or 7 minutes to go in my bottle. We headed out to change our bottles, and when we were heading back up the driveway to go back in through the kitchen, I realized there was a tool off the ladder truck that I thought would be helpful in pulling down the ceiling so we could get right to the fire. I was pulling the tool off the truck when the brakes from the engine company truck, which was positioned right behind the ladder truck, let go and pinned me in between both vehicles. My life flashed before my eyes, and there I was pinned in between. I started screaming.

The chief arrived and ordered someone up into the engine to back it up. Once that happened, the chief was right there. He was holding me. My legs were like Jell-O. I could feel them completely crushed.

I went into the operating room at about 3:30 a.m. The next thing I remember was waking up on Thursday with a breathing tube in my mouth and not knowing what day it was and what had happened. My wife told me that they had to amputate my leg to save my life. Then that's when all the recovery began.

Chapter 12

Harness Your Spiritual Energy

When I was going through cancer treatment, people often asked what they could do for me. Even some of those closest to me were surprised when I said, "Pray for me every night at 9:00 p.m. eastern standard time." Many took my request seriously, even passing it along to their relatives and friends. I know this because people wrote to me to say that they were praying for me every evening. One woman whom I have never met—the mother-in-law of a friend who manages the center where I work—wrote that she was praying for me at 9 o'clock every night and also throughout the day.

Not everyone responded so supportively, however. Some people thought that I was kidding or that my illness had prompted me to do something completely out of character. After all, a doctor at Harvard Medical School is supposed to be more science-minded. Perhaps if I had said simply, "Pray for me," people would have not thought my request so odd. I wanted concentrated prayers at a specific time of day. What was I thinking?

During chemotherapy, 9 o'clock at night was a particularly difficult and lonely time for me. My husband and I would have finished putting all of our children to bed and spent the previous half hour or so talking to each other before I turned in. By 9:00 p.m., I would be in bed—exhausted and usually in pain—and the house would be quiet. Before I would drift off, I would pray, just as has been my custom for more years than I can recall.

As I prayed, I knew that I was helping myself to heal, both physically and emotionally. I've read the studies, and I know that the evidence of the positive health effects of spiritual practice is quite convincing. Whether this therapeutic power is driven by an external force such as divine intervention or by the internal mechanisms of the body is beyond the scope of my expertise. I don't know the answer, and science has yet to reveal one. What I can say with conviction is that for whatever reason, tapping into your own spiritual reservoir—as it feels comfortable for you—can help you to Super Heal.

The word *health* is derived from the Anglican word *hal*, which means "to be whole or holy." Though there are many ways to use spirituality as a healing resource, all spiritual journeys involve quieting the mind and establishing a stronger connection to nature, God or some other deity, or an energy source.

Talking to God

I can't recall a time when I haven't prayed. As a child, I developed the habit of praying before I fall asleep, and my prayers always have a certain order to them. This order comes from a memoir called *I Am Third,* which I read in middle school. The book was written by Gale Sayers, one of the greatest running backs in the history of professional football. It describes Sayers's ascent out of the ghetto and into the national spotlight of pro sports and eventually the Hall of Fame. The title of his book comes from his spiritual philosophy: "The Lord is first; my family and friends are second; I am third." The concept of "I am third" resonated with me, and I have used it ever since as the order in which to pray. Both praying and the order of my prayers is a ritual that comforts me and makes sense to me.

Scientific studies have shown that when people pray, it has positive physical consequences for their health. Intercessory prayer—praying for others—is more controversial. The research into whether others can pray for you and alter the outcome of your medical condition is inconclusive at this time. Some studies seem to suggest that intercessory prayer can help, while others suggest that it doesn't make much difference.

So with no definitive proof of the therapeutic power of prayer and the scientific evidence somewhat contradictory, why would I ask those around me to pray for me at 9 o'clock each night?

I did this for a couple of reasons. First, as I mentioned earlier, I felt acutely alone and vulnerable at this hour. It comforted me immensely to know that so many people cared enough about me to pray for me at the appointed time. Many of my relatives and good friends live in California, where I grew up. This meant that they would pray for me at 6:00 p.m. Pacific standard time, usually a busy hour for most people. The fact that my loved ones would put their lives on hold and pray for me on a daily basis meant much more to me than any gift they could have sent.

A second reason for requesting evening prayers is that I believed they could work in my favor. One scientific explanation for how prayer or meditation can benefit us physically is that it may enhance relaxation and the sense of control, which can directly affect blood pressure and other physiologic parameters. It's possible, too, that spiritual practices—especially those associated with formalized religion—may correlate with better health practices such as not smoking, not drinking excessively, exercising regularly, and eating healthfully.

Of course, the other explanation for how spirituality and religion support physical healing is divine intervention through the direct hand of God or some other higher power. Does God listen to our prayers? There is a story that when Bill Moyers was a special assistant to then president Lyndon B. Johnson, he was asked to say grace prior to a meal in the family's quarters. As Moyers quietly began, the president interrupted him and said, "Speak up, Bill!" Without looking up, Moyers—a former Baptist minister from Texas—promptly replied, "I wasn't addressing you, Mr. President."

Whether or not God listens to prayers is the subject of much debate. At this time, we have no way to scientifically evaluate or validate such a theory. Those who believe in the therapeutic power of divine intervention do so out of faith. What is not nearly so controversial is what medical doctor, Larry Dossey, MD, states in the title of one of his books: *Prayer Is Good Medicine*.

Defining Spirituality, Religion, and Prayer

Spiritual scholars have come up with various definitions to help distinguish between religion and spirituality. Often spirituality is defined as that which is sacred or holy, coupled with a transcendent (greater than self) relationship with God or another higher power or with a universal energy. A panel of experts convened by the National Institute of Healthcare Research defined spirituality as "the feelings, thoughts, experiences, and behaviors that arise from a search for the sacred."

Religion, on the other hand, is more formal. It involves a specific set of beliefs, rituals, and practices that often are culturally ingrained. Spirituality is amorphous, whereas religion has borders and definition. The book *Spirituality and Healing: A Multicultural Perspective* describes religion as "a compilation of beliefs and values through which individuals might relate to spirituality. These beliefs are codified and accepted by members of the religious community. Ideally, religion provides a reliable structure for spiritual practice. Yet by institutionalizing spiritual experience, religions may tend to objectify and dogmatize spirituality." On the other hand: "Authentic spiritual connectedness is characterized by an aptitude for compassion and morality."

People who are spiritual do not necessarily believe in God or another deity. Instead, they may express their spirituality in other ways, such as through a connectedness with nature. While believing in God is not a prerequisite for a spiritual life, the vast majority of people in the United States (at least 95 percent) do believe in God or a higher spiritual power. In *Who Needs God?* Rabbi Harold Kushner writes:

> There are no atheists in foxholes and few atheists in hospitals. It is not because people are hypocrites, ignoring God when things are going smoothly and suddenly discovering Him and pleading piety when they are in trouble. And it is not just a matter of turning to God out of fear. There are no atheists in foxholes because times like those bring us face to face with our limitations. . . . People have always found God at the limits of their own strength.

Many people believe that God uses physicians and other health care providers to help people heal. In a survey conducted in the southeastern United States, 80 percent of respondents cited a belief that God works through physicians to cure illness. In a separate study conducted in Pakistan, 92 percent of respondents agreed that the healing powers of doctors are gifts from God.

Congregational rabbi Samuel Karff notes that in biblical and rabbinic Judaism, there always have been three partners in the healing of the sick. God is the Ultimate Healer, while a "human agent or partner" facilitates healing. The third partner is the ill person himself. Rabbi Karff explains that in this tradition, "proper self-care begins with a recognition that one cannot be physician to one's self, but the patient remains as an active partner with God and the human healer in responding to illness."

Faith is a belief in something for which there is no proof. Prayer, though usually thought of in a religious context, can be associated with nonreligious aspects of spirituality such as meditation. Of note is that these definitions are the subject of great debate and that many religious scholars make a clear distinction between meditation and prayer. For the purposes of this chapter—which is to encourage you to harness your spiritual energy through whatever means appeals to you—I am combining both religious and nonreligious methods of prayer as a general category. My point is not to suggest that all prayer is the same but, rather, to be inclusive and encourage people from all walks of life to consider prayer as a healing resource.

Science, Spirituality, and Healing

For most of history, nearly all healing was entrenched in the spiritual. The relatively recent evolution of evidence-based medicine has prompted a clearer delineation between faith and science. In drawing this line, experts on both sides argued vehemently for their views.

Today, there seems to be room to compromise—to experience the tremendous benefits of both science and spirituality and "integrate" them into the same healing experience. Religious scholar Martin Marty writes of this changing view, "Theorists, scientists, practitioners, and patients, on one side, have come to be more open to the voices of faith and the spiritual searches for well-being. Meanwhile, on the other side, theologians, religious philosophers, pastors, and ordinary believers, discerning such openness, have grown friendlier to science."

Not everyone is open to the idea that spirituality can or should help people with physical healing. In the book *Heal Thyself: Spirituality, Medicine, and the Distortion of Christianity,* two scholars make their case for the opposing view. The book flap sums up their perspective this way:

> *Heal Thyself* argues that our popular culture's fascination with the health benefits of religion reflects not the renaissance of the world's great religious traditions but the powerful combination of pervasive consumer capitalism and a deeply self-interested individualism. A faith-for-health exchange, say the authors, serves to misrepresent and devalue the true meaning of faith.

I definitely am not suggesting that people in the Healing Zone engage in a "faith-for-health exchange." I happen to be a medical doctor who believes in God. I've held this belief throughout my life, in sickness and in health. But not everyone does, and I respect that. It isn't necessary for people who are sick to embrace faith and "find God" in order to get better.

When I treat people who are ill, I do so assuming that they already have formed their own opinions about spirituality and religion. I further assume that as intelligent individuals seeking information about how best to heal, they want this information presented from a scientific, rather than a philosophical, point of view. Finally—since studies reveal this to be true—I assume that the vast majority of my patients believe in a Creator and that those who don't, consider themselves spiritual in other ways.

These assumptions hold up well for most of my patients. They are most interested in knowing the science behind the relationship between spirituality and physical healing. I suspect that the same is true for most of the people who are reading this book. They want to know what the research shows and will make up their own minds about how to use the information.

As a medical doctor, I believe that it's imperative to share with patients what we know about the science of physical healing. As a person of faith, I want to reassure them that both science and spirituality can coexist in harmony. Professor Marty's work espouses this modern, integrative approach to healing. He writes, "Some of the hostile attitudes of the past may be seen as increasingly limited and obsolete. . . . It would be as unscientific to overlook the insights of faith communities as it may be faithless to fear the effects of science in the healing communities."

To me, it's possible to be both a scientist who is interested in facts and a sincerely spiritual person who understands that some things have yet to be revealed to us. In his book *Belief in God in an Age of Science,* physicist and theologian John Polkinghorne describes how both a strong science background and a strong sense of faith can coexist. He writes, "I believe that nuclear matter is made up of quarks which are not only unseen but which are also invisible in principle (because they are permanently confined within the protons and neutrons they constitute). The effects of these quarks can be perceived, but not the entities themselves. . . . A similar conviction grounds my belief in the invisible reality of God."

The Physical Benefits of Spirituality

The study of how spirituality and physical healing intersect is in its infancy, though the early data quite convincingly point to a significant positive relationship. The research from the field known as psychoneuroimmunology, which I mentioned previously in this book, is especially fascinating. For example, one study found that students who watched a religious movie had a much more positive immune response—as measured by increases in levels of immunoglobulin A, or IgA—than students who watched a war movie. In another study involving 1,700 people, those who regularly attended religious services were more than 40 percent less likely than nonattendees to have high levels of interleukin-6, a marker of inflammation. Still other studies have produced similar results, suggesting that spirituality can influence immune function and healing.

Meanwhile, other research points to a positive relationship between spirituality and physical health that contributes to lower blood pressure, lower blood fats (lipids), and even longer life span. Still, much about this relationship remains a mystery. In a review article titled "Spiritual Role in Healing: An Alternative Way of Thinking," which appeared in the medical journal *Primary Care Clinical Office Practice,* the authors summarized the current state of psychoneuroimmunological research by noting, "The link between religion and health is established firmly. What remains tentative is whether it is causal, and, if so, by which mechanisms does it work? Many possible mechanisms may play a role, such as lower rates of drug and alcohol abuse, improved stress management, and enhanced social support."

One of the pioneers in the field of psychoneuroimmunology is Candace Pert, PhD, a former research professor at Georgetown University School of Medicine in Washington, DC, and section chief at the National Institute of Mental Health. Dr. Pert explains her stance on spirituality and science in this manner:

> I'm a scientist viewing the realm of the spirit, approaching it with hard-core, observable evidence; and from the data I've seen, I can no longer deny the existence of God. . . . In the matter of science and God coming together, I'm in good company with another scientist, one much more famous and influential than myself: Albert Einstein. His professional journey brought him to a personal epiphany in which he proclaimed that the more he understood the universe, the more he believed that a Creator was at work.

Religion and Mood

Back in Chapter 10, I discussed at length the relationship between mood and physical healing. Religion, as it pertains to someone being a member of a community of faith, can confer significant emotional benefits. For example, we know that people who are religious experience less depression, are less likely to abuse drugs or alcohol, are better able to cope with adverse life events, and are less likely to commit suicide. Both in the general population and among those facing serious illness, religion seems to protect against depression—and if a person does become depressed, he's likely to recover more quickly if he's religious than if he's not.

Unfortunately, some people use religion in a destructive manner. You'll find many examples of this throughout ancient and modern history. It stands to reason that when religion serves as a vehicle for persecution or as a shield for committing immoral acts, then it quite possibly is deleterious to the health of the individual and the health of others.

Another way in which religion can result in physical harm is when it's cited as a reason to not seek medical intervention. There are many documented instances of this, such as the case of *McKown v. Lundman*. In this particular case, the Minnesota Court of Appeals awarded $1.5 million to the father of 11-year-old Ian Lundman, who died after his mother, stepfather, and two Christian Science practitioners tried to use prayer to heal his diabetes. Following the Supreme Court's 1996 decision not to review the case, thus upholding the lower court's ruling, the *New York Times* ran an op-ed piece titled "The Power of Prayer Denied."

Such abuses should not detract from the fact that religion and spirituality—when practiced with a keen regard for morality and kindness—can be wonderful resources for a journey through the Healing Zone. In a study titled "Allowing Spirituality into the Healing Process" in the *Journal of Family Practice,* the author summarized the research on the relationship between religion, spirituality, and healing in this manner:

> In general, research shows the impact of religion and spirituality is positive. Although a person's spirituality is sometimes pathological, and spiritual beliefs can create health issues, an overwhelming number of studies show a positive benefit. . . . [In studies] where the impact of spirituality could be classified as positive, negative, no association, complex, or mixed, 70 percent showed a positive impact . . . while only 5 percent showed a negative impact. The studies show spirituality and religion benefit patients by helping prevent illness, increasing the ability to cope, and improving outcomes.

Richard Materson, MD, is a doctor who—like myself—has trained in rehabilitation medicine. He also is an advocate of spirituality and healing. Though his interest in this topic began many years ago, it was in 2002—when he collapsed during a medical conference and was rushed to the hospital—that his spiritual and physical healing journeys intersected in a profound and life-changing way. "Dick" Materson, who was one of the doctors who trained me, lived through an illness that usually claims nearly all of its victims. You'll read his Remarkable Recovery story on page 199. Though Dr. Materson's journey through the Healing Zone was long and arduous, he healed optimally and has served on the board of the Institute for Religion and Health of the Texas Medical Center in Houston.

The Power of Prayer

Religion, in its most advantageous form to support healing, often enhances spirituality through formal rituals and practices. Francis MacNutt has written several books on prayer and healing from a Christian perspective. In *The Power to Heal,* he describes the Sacrament of the Sick, noting that this ritual helps to "build up the faith" of the ill person and assist her in spending time praying.

But formal religion definitely is not the only way in which people can tap into the healing power of spirituality. Prayer—which can be as simple as a single sentence that you don't even need to utter aloud (e.g., "Please, God, give me strength")—is a terrific tool that you can access whenever you need it.

In his book *Getting Through What You're Going Through*, Rev. Robert Anthony Schuller writes about how it is good to look back at what has already happened in your life and to draw on those memories during turbulent times. Rev. Schuller offers this thoughtful advice about prayer: "Remembering how God has guided you through a difficult time is one way to help you get through your going through stage. Your prayer should be, 'Guide me, Lord. Guide me again, as you did before.'"

When it comes to prayer, some people aren't sure where or how to begin. The nice thing about it is that there's no "right" way to do it. Any way you want to pray will be just fine. If you prefer a nonreligious context, consider using meditation as your method of prayer.

Sasha Kondratiuk, the young assault victim whose story I've revisited on several occasions over the course of this book, received many prayers from others but had trouble praying on her own. In her words, she describes how she handled this aspect of her recovery.

> I am Ukrainian Orthodox, and it was really wonderful that the priest in Washington came to visit me in the hospital almost every day to pray with my family and me. I really appreciated it, and I think it did strengthen my mental state and calm me. In a colder and more practical sense, I think prayer also made me feel better to the extent that I was covering all my bases in terms of healing. Many people sent me healing oils that were blessed from around the world, and I used those. I also knew that so many people were praying for me and holding religious services for me, which also made me feel better.
>
> On my own, however, I found it difficult to pray when I was alone, since I was so blown away by everything that was happening. I suppose I couldn't really wrap my head around why something so horrible could happen to me, and therefore, I felt like it was somewhat useless to pray since it probably wouldn't really make a difference anyway.

While praying regularly is an excellent way to tap into your spirituality, it isn't your only option. For example, simply taking a walk outside where you can enjoy nature is soothing and relaxing for your mind and body. Almost everyone who takes the time to sit in a beautiful place—whether it's near the ocean, in the woods, on a park bench, or anywhere else that is peaceful and serene—will be able to utilize this experience spiritually. The world is a magnificent place; use it to support your recovery.

If you are more adventurous and you're able to, explore other activities with a spiritual component. For example, one journalist who interviewed me for a story on breast cancer told me that when she was recovering from cancer treatment herself, she decided to train to climb a mountain in Colorado. She described both the training and the actual climb in a very spiritual context—one that involved connecting with nature and a higher power. I have talked with many other people in various stages of illness and recovery who have planned spiritual vacations to India, Israel, Rome, and other wonderful places.

Scaling a mountain or traveling to the Vatican can be incredibly fulfilling, but so can enjoying the spiritual opportunities that present themselves on a daily basis. For example, one day I was meeting friends for dinner in Boston's North End (the city's Italian section). As we were walking to the restaurant, we passed a beautiful historic Catholic church. On the spur of the moment, we decided to go inside. The church's architecture and stained-glass windows combined with hundreds of candles flickering in the semidarkness were just breathtaking. My friends and I knelt, prayed silently, and then left feeling very much at peace.

Peace often is lacking when you travel through the Healing Zone. Tapping into your spirituality offers you a respite from turmoil.

Promoting Spirituality and Loving Connections in Your Family

I wasn't the only one who needed a respite from the turmoil that my cancer caused. My loved ones needed a break, too—which is why I talked with our parish priest, Father Jim Houston, about how to gently encourage spirituality in my children. As an avid reader himself, he often recommended books to his parishioners. For me he selected one called *Raising Faith-Filled Kids*. A number of messages in this book resonated with me; I'll share two of them with you.

One is that rituals help to instill and promote spirituality. This is true for adults as well as for children. Our family has a lot of rituals that I doubt my children even recognize as such. Instead, they are part of the intricate threads that make up the fabric of our daily lives.

One of our rituals is to say grace before dinner. As Catholics, we first make the sign of the cross, and then—in our version of this ritual—we join hands. Usually we say a formal prayer that starts out with the words "Bless us, O Lord, and these your gifts . . . " For my children, this prayer has special meaning. It is said at all of the family dinners on my husband's side. My husband's parents, his seven siblings, their spouses, and their children recite this prayer when they're together. In our home, we usually share this ritual with just our immediate family, though we also offer it whenever we have guests for dinner.

For my children, this ritual is extremely meaningful, though I assume that at this point in their young lives, they don't realize the full impact. Do you remember the "12 points of connection" from the previous chapter? The first point is to connect with your family of origin. My children often say this prayer in unison with their extended family, including their grandparents, aunts, uncles, and cousins. The second point is to connect with your immediate family, which this ritual does both literally (as we hold hands) and figuratively. The fourth point is to connect with friends; when our cherished friends join us around the table, we invite them to say this prayer with us. The sixth point is to connect with the past, and certainly the practice of Catholicism is deeply rooted in my children's ancestry—especially through their paternal grandmother, whose family emigrated from Ireland to the United States. Finally, saying grace connects my children to the 11th point—whatever is beyond knowledge, or spirituality.

So with this one ritual, my children engage in five of the 12 points of connection identified by psychiatrist Edward Hallowell, MD. Though I started this particular ritual long before I read Dr. Hallowell's list, it's fascinating to see how spirituality and connection can be so powerfully intertwined.

A ritual can be whatever feels comfortable for you and your family. It is the process of doing something over and over that brings comfort, reassurance, and peace. Rituals can include giving thanks before a meal, attending a religious service, celebrating a spiritual holiday, going to a special place on a regular basis to commune with nature, volunteering in a soup kitchen, and so on. There are so many valuable rituals to include in your spiritual quest.

The second message that resonated with me was the use of symbols in the home. Formal religions often have beautiful symbols that help to remind people of their connection to a particular faith, but other things can also remind us of our connection to the larger world and especially to nature. A stunning stone or piece of wood, a painting of a majestic place, or a colorful fish tank can help to soothe and connect us.

Harnessing Your Spiritual Energy to Help You Heal

I decided to include a chapter on spirituality because the scientific evidence to support the positive effects on health and healing is so compelling. Perhaps you already are using spiritual energy, in the form of prayer or another technique, to support the healing process.

I do recommend setting both short- and long-term spiritual goals while you're in the Healing Zone. Whether or not you do so is your choice. If you do, you might want to review the ideas for goals on page 198. These are meant to facilitate healing for anyone, regardless of personal philosophy or belief system.

The research in this area of medicine does not support or endorse any one type of spirituality or religion over another. I doubt it ever will. My husband once told me this joke, which I think highlights how ridiculous it would be for a higher power to choose sides.

> *The head football coach at USC, Pete Carroll, and the head foot-ball coach at Notre Dame, Charlie Weis, both die and go to heaven. After they pass through the pearly gates, God greets them and shows them to their new homes. God takes Carroll to a nice but slightly older house with "USC" painted on the door. The yard is small but well kept. Carroll is pleased until he looks next door and sees an enormous, newly constructed mansion painted entirely in Notre Dame's colors, blue and gold. The immense lawn is as beautifully landscaped as any park. Out front there is a solid gold flagpole, 50 feet tall, with a magnifi-cent banner bearing the crest of the University of Notre Dame.*
>
> *Carroll says: "God, I hate to seem ungrateful, but why do I get an ordinary house while Weis gets that luxurious palace?"*
>
> *God replies: "That's not Weis's house—that's mine."*

As a Notre Dame alum, my husband would prefer for God to side with his team during football season. But I can't imagine a God who would choose sides, whether in football or in healing. Moreover, the science cer-tainly does not support this concept. Thus, I am not advocating any par-ticular religion or practice, but I do encourage you to consider the body of scientific evidence that illustrates the positive effects of spirituality on healing.

Of course, as a medical doctor, I would never advise anyone to rely solely on prayer or other spiritual connections as a method of healing. My suggestion to those who are spiritual is to use this energy or power in conjunction with proven medical treatments.

I know that everyone who reads this chapter—including you—will have their own personal philosophies about religion and spirituality and about the true nature of the positive relationship between spirituality and healing. Some may believe that it all boils down to science and the complex biochemical reactions that connect mind and body. Others may feel that divine intervention is the only plausible explanation. But the majority, I suspect, share a more middle-of-the-road view in which both science and spirituality play a role.

Short- and Long-Term Spiritual Goals

Much like your love goals, your spiritual goals are intensely personal. I offer the following to you simply to get you thinking about what your goals might be. Choose those that feel comfortable to you.

Short-Term

- Make time to pray alone once a day.
- Add a family prayer before one meal a day.
- Listen to religious music once a week.
- Commune with nature for 30 minutes once a week.
- Attend a religious ceremony (e.g., a service, wedding, or baptism) once during the month.
- Make an appointment to meet with a priest, minister, rabbi, or spiritual counselor of your choosing.
- Add a religious symbol that brings you comfort to a favorite place in your home.
- Spend 15 minutes a day reading the Bible, Talmud, Koran, or other great religious tome.
- Read a book on the topic of spirituality. Choose one that offers a hopeful, uplifting message.
- Engage in some type of community service, such as volunteering at a soup kitchen or shelter.

Long-Term

- Attend religious services as regularly as possible.
- Celebrate religious holidays in new and meaningful ways.
- Continue daily prayers.
- Plan a spiritual vacation that may include meditation, prayer, visiting spiritually significant places, or communing with nature.
- Make a plan to read the entire Bible or another great religious text during the year.

Rabbi Karff is of this latter mind-set. As he explains:

> I believe that God heals through ministrations of a good physician or the biochemical fruits of scientific research, and I account these researchers and physicians as God's designated partners in healing. I also believe God may, and sometimes does, heal independently, and that such healing may be in response to prayer. In other words, God's power to heal the body is not simply reducible to the intervention of physicians, surgeons, and drugs.

Paul Eustace—whose son sustained a devastating injury after being struck by an out-of-control car—called me one day and said, "I want to tell you about the people who prayed for David." Paul, who was overwhelmed with grief and kept a constant bedside vigil for his son, didn't realize until many months later that a vast network of people was asking God to help heal David. Paul told me that one group started at his church and met regularly to pray for his child. They, in turn, asked members of other churches to pray. Paul learned that prayer groups as far away as England were including his son in their conversations with God. Paul said, "There is a boy downstairs right now who is playing with David. This child prayed every day for my child." Paul went on to say that he couldn't discount the possibility that prayers somehow contributed to David's recovery—and to saving his life.

On a Sunday just prior to Thanksgiving, I went to Mass and was listening to my parish priest deliver a sermon on thanks and gratitude. Father Houston—who often quotes people of various religious backgrounds—cited the legendary evangelical minister Dwight Lyman Moody, who is given credit for saying, "We pray like it is all up to God, and we work like it is all up to us." Then and there, I realized that this is the closing message I want for this chapter: Pray that you'll heal as well as possible, and at the same time, work to recover optimally. Whether or not you believe in divine intervention, science is on your side.

REMARKABLE RECOVERY

Richard Materson

In the fall of 2002, I was in Orlando, Florida, for the American Academy of Physical Medicine and Rehabilitation meeting, and I was giving a lecture. The night before, I hadn't slept very well. I had had a wound on my foot patched over with a graft by my doctor just before I left. What I didn't realize was that it was probably infected.

To make a long story short, I felt funny during the talk and asked one of my former residents to take me out of the room. He was able to get me to the lobby of the convention center and put me on a couch, where I promptly lost consciousness. At the hospital they diagnosed me with acute respiratory distress syndrome, called ARDS, which has about a 90 percent fatality rate. My wife was there with me, and they told her and the rest of my family to get a black suit and a box because I wasn't going home.

Well, strange things happen. Lee Kaiser, who has my personal vote for one of the most productive people on earth in the movement of humanistic holistic medicine, happened to be there. He's a Seventh Day Adventist clergyman as well, an elder in that church. When he heard I had been admitted, he came to my bedside—apparently at the time that I was at my worst—and stayed and just prayed quietly over me. I was unconscious, but my wife later told me that the power of that prayer was unbelievable—not just in the kindness of it but, she thought, perhaps in the effect, too. One never knows. Then outside of my room he had a group of 300 Adventists, who did some intercessory praying for me as well.

Later I was transferred to the Texas Institute for Rehabilitation and Research. I was out of it mentally until I woke up about 6 weeks later in the brain injury unit, having sustained a lack of enough oxygen to the brain. By the time I woke up, my muscles had atrophied so that I could hardly pick a limb off the bed. With good rehabilitation techniques, I eventually was able to go home. I now can take a few steps but mostly use a power scooter.

I had been introduced to the board of the Institute for Religion and Health at the Texas Medical Center. The board was made up half of interfaith clergy and half of health professionals and community leaders. Some very prominent Houstonians who wanted to see growth of the ethical and spiritual and compassionate had founded it about 50 years ago as part of the Texas Medical Center—a center known for its biomedical and scientific excellence. Eventually, I was elected chair of the board.

In the group, of course, are many clergy. It was interesting, because they all wanted to know if I had seen the light and crossed the bridge when I had my illness. I think they were a little disappointed that I was unconscious or couldn't remember. But they were enormously supportive.

These are people of all faiths. Whether they're religious or not, they're there to assist and to do the things that a spiritual community does for its friends and colleagues when they're hurt. And that support is just inestimable in getting you to think positively and to improve. I did pray for myself, and I accepted with a great deal of gratitude the prayers of people who were of every religion. They were all, as far as I can tell, given not to proselytize or to influence anything except a good recovery.

I am absolutely convinced by my study of this area that we're at the very pioneer level of understanding brain chemistry, recovery, the healing process, all of those things. And while medicine is chipping away at it, real good is being done by people who perhaps don't know the physiology of what their things are doing—the meditation, the yoga, the tai chi, the healing touch, just holding somebody's hand and squeezing it when you're a nurse at the bedside. Those things have powerful healing effects that we're learning about now.

PART 3

Fine-Tuning Your Super Healing Plan

Chapter 13

Revisit Your Goals and Persevere

In the fall of 2005, almost exactly 2 years after my breast cancer diagnosis, I participated in a fund-raising walk in Boston for the Susan G. Komen Foundation. This is a 5-K (3.1-mile) course, and though I didn't time myself, it probably took me less than 45 minutes to reach the finish line. My husband went with me and ran the course in approximately half that time.

Later I would learn that among the 6,000 or more participants was a woman who had been in a serious car accident the previous year. Together with her husband and a very pregnant friend who walked with her, Noorul Rahman completed the course in just over 2 hours. It was the 12th time that she had participated in this charitable event, but on each previous occasion she had run it. This time, she was the last to cross the finish line. It didn't matter. Simply completing this 5-K walk, no matter how long it took, was one of Noorul's goals.

Two months later, Noorul became one of my patients. As she explains, the accident changed her life dramatically.

> Before the accident, I was a very avid runner. I set a goal with a friend of mine to run one race every month, and we did. My goal for 2005 was to run the Boston Marathon with a co-worker, to raise money for Dana-Farber Cancer Institute. I was very physical, very active. After the accident, I could barely walk. I still am having some problems with balance.

At the time Noorul came to see me, she was on the cusp of the 1-year anniversary of her accident. She had healed quite a bit, but she was determined to achieve more. (Her Remarkable Recovery story appears at the end of this chapter.)

Throughout Noorul's recovery, I have encouraged her to set goals and revisit them. She is an extremely accomplished person, with a PhD in chemistry, and a self-described workaholic. She has always thrived on setting and achieving goals, and she still has a tendency to "shoot for the moon." One of Noorul's goals is to again run the Komen course in Boston. I am not sure if it's realistic for her. I've advised her to keep this goal tucked in her mind while she concentrates on short- and long-term goals that she can achieve within a recovery-based time frame (4 weeks for short-term, 6 months for long-term).

This has been difficult for Noorul. She always has had very high expectations for herself and, generally, has been able to meet them. Now she must be satisfied with accomplishing less than what she wants. It hasn't been easy, but she does it with grace. In short, she perseveres.

As Noorul's doctor, I walk a fine line between wanting to encourage her and help her remain hopeful but also understanding the importance of steering her toward realistic goals. Goals that are out of reach tend to discourage people and hamper healing.

Setting goals is a process that requires constant revisiting. It's impossible to know at the outset exactly how much you can accomplish in a few weeks or months. Author Henriette Klauser gives a great example of how a real journey needs constant attention to stay on course. She writes:

> A plane flying from the mainland to Hawaii is, 90 percent of the time, off course—but it is constantly correcting. The pilot knows he's headed to Hawaii, so when the plane deviates, or the wind throws him off course, he checks his needle and magnetic heading, adjusts, and gets back on track. Eventually, the plane lands on that tiny island in a huge ocean—on exactly the right, narrow airstrip. So too with goals, we need to check our compass and remember where we are heading.

Noorul recognizes the importance of goals and the need to regularly reevaluate them. One of her goals was to improve her time in the Komen. As I was writing this chapter, she again was participating in the event. She shaved 20 minutes off her previous time, though she still finished last. Is this failure or success? It depends on how you look at it. I encourage Noorul to consider it a spectacular success. Few people, regardless of their health status, could shave 20 minutes off their race time in 12 months. Noorul has committed herself to healing, and it's paying off.

As you focus on your own recovery, keep in mind the importance of measuring, monitoring, and redefining your goals over time. Revisiting your goals on a monthly basis allows you to set new short-term goals and decide whether your long-term ones still seem appropriate. I hope this is not a chore but, rather, an opportunity to see your progress and thus maintain your motivation. It's a process that helps you to persevere.

Perseverance

A dictionary definition of *persevere* is "to persist in a state, enterprise, or undertaking in spite of counterinfluences, opposition, or discouragement." I once took a college course for which Dave Scott was a guest lecturer. What I remember most from his talk was his comment that he never had been a stellar athlete. He rarely took first place in any of the athletic events in which he competed. But he noticed that during practices, he seemed to last longer than anyone else. He had more endurance than his teammates, as well as his competitors. He was better able to persevere.

Scott decided to take advantage of his perseverance by training for and competing in triathlons. He achieved astounding success, becoming a six-time Ironman World Champion. (If you're not familiar with it, the Ironman is a 2-day event in Hawaii that consists of a 2.4-mile swim, 112-mile bike ride, and 26.2-mile marathon.) Not surprisingly, Scott became the most recognized athlete in the sport of triathlon and was the first inductee into the Ironman Hall of Fame.

Perseverance doesn't mean that you are happy-go-lucky. The Healing Zone is a tough place to be, and it's normal to occasionally feel discouraged while you're there. Noorul tells me that she has a daily "pity party" for herself, and then she gets on with what she needs to do. Noorul, accustomed to flashy success in her career and her personal life, has needed to readjust her expectations. Helen Keller, an icon of perseverance and success, once summed it up this way: "I long to accomplish a great and noble task, but it is my chief duty to accomplish small tasks as if they were great and noble." In the Healing Zone, it's the small tasks that add up, and even if they don't seem like a big deal at the time, they move you closer to your goal of physical recovery.

So many people throughout history have achieved success solely because of their unwavering perseverance. As humorist Doc Blakey once said, "Success is getting up just one more time than you fall down." Both Abraham Lincoln and Winston Churchill are notorious for their many, many failures early in their careers. Churchill had experienced a lifetime of adversity before finally becoming prime minister of England at age 62—then considered a senior citizen. As a world leader, he personified perseverance, rallying the spirit and resolve of a nation as it faced the superior

German forces in World War II. In his later years, Churchill was invited to address the graduating class at Oxford University. The audience hushed as he walked up to the podium, said five words, and then sat down again. His simple message to those students still resonates today: "Never, never, never give up."

Trusting Your Body Again

A key element of persevering is learning to trust your body again. In Chapter 5, I shared the story of snowboarder Chris Klug, who won a bronze medal at the Winter Olympics just 18 months after undergoing a liver transplant. What is remarkable about Klug is not only his amazing athletic prowess but also his incredible ability to heal. Klug is a fierce competitor and is thrilling to watch in action, but the most incredible part of his story is his journey from transplant patient to Olympic champion.

Just 7 weeks after his transplant, Klug returned to snowboarding. He told me, "At first the doctor had me on a pretty tight leash, but I felt like a new engine got dropped in me. I just knew I was going to make it back." But he also tells of how he worried that if he crashed, his very extensive surgical wound could open up. In his memoir *To the Edge and Back,* he wrote, "Driving up to the ski area, I experienced a mixture of eagerness and fear. I was excited to be back, but I was also afraid. *What if I fall?* Would I literally burst open at the purple seam that stretched across my abdomen? Might some organ tear loose or twist inside me, and I wouldn't know it until I wound up in a hospital again?"

Learning to trust his body again was a major obstacle that Klug needed to overcome in order to realize his lifetime goal of becoming an Olympic champion. I asked physical therapist and sports trainer Bill Fabrocini how he was able to help Klug over this hurdle. Fabrocini explained that he started by setting small goals to build Klug's confidence without stressing the injury. He told me, "I did a lot of working around the injury—all the other segments of his body. I wanted Chris to think positively about the uninjured areas and to focus on what was working well. Then I connected all of the areas together so that the body started to [function] as a whole. That is what breeds confidence."

For all serious athletes, physical goal setting is central to their training. To go faster, jump higher, or improve accuracy is all-important. Klug was able to Super Heal because he invested his time and energy in healing and because he set goals and adjusted them as he went along.

Today when Klug gives motivational speeches, he talks about both his tremendous sports career and his journey through the Healing Zone. He shared with me part of his message to his audiences.

I was in the 11th hour of the transplant waiting process. When I got to that 11th hour, I started to lose hope. I knew the realities of it. But at the same time, I kept pushing forward. I was on the transplant list for 6 years total and for 3 months at the critical stage. I couldn't even play golf; I was pretty wrecked. I would go to the gym and cheer my brother and my buddies on, thinking that maybe I got some benefit just by being there. . . . I like to talk about my two great races—my snowboard race and my race for life.

In both of his "great races," Klug faced many challenges. Through it all, he maintained his faith in himself, and he persevered. He learned to trust his body again, and he adjusted his goals as he went along. Neither his journey through the Healing Zone nor his quest to become an Olympic champion was flawless. In fact, he told me, "When I won my bronze medal in the Olympics, I broke my boot and duct-taped it. I learned I had to make do."

As you assess and adjust your goals, you might follow Klug's lead by adopting more of a whole-body perspective to physical healing. Sometimes it helps to shift the focus of your goals from mending the problem areas to further strengthening what already is working well.

Don't Overfocus on One Part of the Plan

Over time, you may consciously or subconsciously pay attention to some goals more than others. This isn't necessarily a problem, but I encourage you to consider all of the components of the Super Healing Plan. Focusing too much on one or two can impede your ability to heal optimally.

An article in *Newsweek* titled "Healing War's Wounds" highlighted the importance of comprehensive rehabilitation care for injured combat veterans. As I mentioned in Chapter 1, the specialty of physical medicine and rehabilitation (PM&R)—which espouses a multidisciplinary, comprehensive-care approach to healing—began in response to the needs of injured World War II veterans. Despite more sophisticated and destructive weapons, our ability to save the lives of those who serve our country is improving. According to the article, "Thanks to advances in combat medicine and body armor, more than 90 percent of the 20,000 US forces wounded to date in Iraq and Afghanistan are surviving their injuries. (In Vietnam, that figure was closer to 75 percent.)"

Military doctors—some of whom are my colleagues in physiatry, specializing in rehabilitation medicine—increasingly recognize the need for injured soldiers to have a Super Healing Plan. Though they don't call it that, they utilize similar concepts to help their patients recover optimally. The *Newsweek* article reports that the military has "adopted a holistic mind-body approach, deploying a fleet of experts ranging from orthopedic surgeons to therapists to work on the wounded." That's exactly what is needed for soldiers, and anyone else, facing serious illness or injury. As Lt. Col. John McManus notes in the article, "Technology has advanced to the point where we can salvage patients who would not have survived before . . . [but] can we restore a life worth living?"

While you may be tempted to focus on just those goals directly linked to physical recovery (e.g., exercise), remember that the mind-body connection is equally important to healing. In fact, it has become such an essential and recognized component of the healing process that even in the macho military world—where, for instance, love and nurturing tend to be in short supply—health care professionals who are members of the armed forces are introducing mind-body principles into their rehabilitation programs. As you revisit your goals, consider how all of them interconnect with each other and how optimal healing can occur when you focus on all of the components of the Super Healing Plan.

It's common for people to use military terms—like "fight," "battle," and "win"—when they're facing illness or injury. Sometimes such analogies apply to the healing process itself. The great Russian military commander Georgi Zhukov said, "It is a fact that under equal conditions, large-scale battles and whole wars are won by troops which have a strong will for victory, clear goals before them, high moral standards, and devotion to the banner under which they go into battle." I could say something similar about people who heal optimally: They have a strong desire to heal, clear goals before them, the capacity to nurture themselves and others, and a devotion to the idea that, despite setbacks and plateaus, they can persevere.

Batting .500 Will Get You into the Hall of Fame

Professional baseball players who get a hit in roughly half of their at-bats—in other words, they're batting .500—are shoo-ins for the Hall of Fame. Of course, if you follow baseball, you know that no player ever has achieved such an incredible batting average. Instead, Hall of Fame players are more likely to get a hit on every third at-bat. Die-hard baseball fans, while rooting for their home teams, respect the individual players. They know that these men will have more misses than hits in their careers, but still they are great athletes.

Super Healing is a lot like baseball. There will be hits and misses, moments of glory and moments of disappointment. If you want to get into the Super Healing Hall of Fame, here's what you need to do.

Aim to bat .500. If you accomplish half of your goals, you are doing great. Congratulate and reward yourself. But even if you meet only a couple of your goals each month, you still are making progress, and you still could enter the Hall of Fame. Don't let striking out a few times deter you. It's just part of the process.

Educate yourself continuously. After you read this book, continue to educate yourself about how you can best heal. Your doctor can help. Talk with him or her about your goals and your path to optimal recovery.

Create new goals each month, without fail. Schedule time in your calendar and go someplace peaceful and nurturing, such as a local park or beach. Reflect on your progress toward your goals, and reward yourself for all your hard work. As you review your goals, you might want to keep the same one in a particular category if you didn't achieve it because you just didn't spend enough time on it. On the other hand, if you did devote time to it but weren't able to accomplish it, then you might revise the goal or create a new one. Just be kind to yourself as you go through this process.

Move the chain. I teach a course for doctors on how to publish books. One doctor, who has become a dear friend, took my course and then came back the following year to speak to attendees about her progress over the previous 12 months. I am sure that the audience expected her to say that she had published a book and was well on her way to becoming a successful author. But that isn't what she told them. Instead she said, "I'm moving the chain." With this football analogy, she meant that while her ultimate goal is to publish a book (equivalent to a touchdown), she is proceeding step-by-step (or yard by yard)—writing articles for newspapers, magazines, and Web sites to build up her credentials.

If you've watched football, you likely have noticed that the sideline officials move the chain forward as the offensive team gains yardage. "Moving the chain" simply is a process that gets you to where you want to be. In order to Super Heal, all you need to do is keep moving the chain.

Persevere. Many people already have earned their places in the Super Healing Hall of Fame. You probably know some of them personally. Instead of asking for an autograph, ask how they did it. What helped them to persevere? Perseverance is your ticket to optimal recovery.

Looking Back, Looking Forward

Committing yourself to checking your goals, recording your progress, and revising goals as necessary is essential to advancing through the Healing Zone. In the next chapter, I'll talk about how to anticipate and overcome any setbacks and plateaus you may encounter on your healing journey. This is very helpful as you evaluate your goals and consider whether to change or replace them.

Keep in mind that in all of life's challenges, it is those who persevere who have the greatest ability to accomplish what they set out to do. President Ulysses S. Grant summed it up in this way: "In every battle there comes a time when both sides consider themselves beaten. Then he who continues the attack wins."

REMARKABLE RECOVERY

Noorulhuda Rahman

My adventure began on December 17, 2004. I have no recollection of the day of the accident itself. From what I've been told, on my way to work, a truck driver who was not trained to drive a truck with a bobcat attached to it lost control and basically T-boned into my car. They initially called it a fatality accident. It took 45 minutes to extricate me from the car. The rescue crew thought that I was dead, but when they actually cut my seat belt, I started gasping for air. It took them about another half hour to be able to intubate me so I could get some oxygen.

I remember being in the rehabilitation hospital in February, and I didn't know why I was there. Nobody actually told me why I was there. My first reaction was that I was being involuntarily held in the hospital and I wanted to leave. I thought the only way that I could do that was by calling the police and telling them that I was being held involuntarily. I was delusional, obviously.

It was actually about 2 weeks after I was discharged from the hospital that I saw my primary care physician. My husband, Tom, was with me, and they were discussing what the issues were. That was when I found out about my traumatic brain injury. I think at that point in time I did not get a sense for how bad the accident was. Whenever Tom talked about it, he talked about how bad it was. I thought he was overly emotional and it can't be that bad.

Tom actually went to the garage where they hauled my car, because they had all my personal belongings that I had to claim. He took pictures of the car, but he doesn't want me to see them yet because he doesn't think I'm ready for it. I just get a sense it's prob-ably harder for him because . . . well, he didn't know if I was going to make it, because for the first 2 weeks that I was at Mass Memorial, they didn't know if I was going to make it. In fact, when I went back for my hematoma surgery, the people who cared for me the first 2 weeks I was there said, "We are really surprised that you're still here. We really didn't think you were going to make it through."

If you look at me, there's really nothing physical that you can see wrong with me. But I had bleeding in my brain, and I had to go through brain surgery to drain it about 6 months after I got discharged from the hospital. The biggest manifestation of the accident is a traumatic brain injury. You know how on the computer if you don't do a good reboot of the computer, you go through all these different problems? It's not necessarily that everything went bad; it's just sections having "file not found" kind of issues.

Now I'm going through rehab, basically just trying to get my life back to some semblance of normalcy. I'd like to kid myself into thinking that things will get back to normal. It's hard because in a way I feel like I'm an overachiever. To me, to get a B is a failing grade, you know? And I think the biggest failure you can have is when you fail in your goals.

I've always set goals for myself. I tried to make sure I graduated with my BS before I turned 21, and I did. I wanted to make sure that I graduated with my PhD before I turned 35, and I did. I wanted to buy a house before 30, and I did. My next goal was to be a vice president in a company before I turned 45, and now I feel like that is at risk. I don't know.

To me, not attaining your goals is what comprises a failure. If I don't make vice president before I'm 45, then that will the first real failure in life. I'm not optimistic. I'm trying to be realistic so that I won't be completely discouraged.

My darkest hour was when I first realized that this was almost a fatal accident. That was a hard thing to reconcile. And, of course, the second darkest hour was when I started to realize that I might not be able to achieve my goals. I'm 43. It's never happened before. And now having to learn to deal with that at this age—it's tough.

My husband is my rock. I mean, I never thought anyone would be able to give me the kind of support that I get from him. It's just beyond what I would ever expect. For example, when I first was discharged from the hospital, and I had to go to the bathroom, he would carry me and put me on the toilet. He would make sure that I cleaned myself well and then carried me back.

Just recently he was downstairs on the phone and I was taking a shower. As I was stepping out of the shower, I actually fell, and he heard me fall from downstairs. He came running up and he was there in a jiff, like almost instantly there. And I thought, "How did he do that?" But he would put everything, his career and everything, aside to make sure that I'm comfortable. So now he hauls me everywhere he goes; he travels a lot for his work, and he makes sure that I go with him. From my perspective, I'm an added burden, but you would never hear him say that. He's been my rock, yes. I see the strength in him that I otherwise would never see.

Chapter 14

Cope with Setbacks and Plateaus

"**N**ext week there can't be any crisis. My schedule is already full."
Henry Kissinger said this in jest, but wouldn't it be great if we really could clear our schedules of disruptions and just focus on healing? It would be even better if healing occurred exponentially or even linearly in an upward slope—all forward progress, with no dips or blips to discourage us.

But just as Kissinger couldn't avoid dealing with constant governmental crises, we can't heal without facing hurdles, stumbling blocks, and even reversals. This is because normal healing involves setbacks and plateaus. For Super Healing, then, you need to be able to navigate these situations without letting them throw you completely off course.

Doctors are very familiar with the idea that healing is not a linear process, flowing smoothly from start to finish. In fact, they constantly are helping patients overcome detours in their progress. Because doctors anticipate these sorts of challenges, however, they may not recognize how discouraged patients feel when they encounter one. What doctors take for granted and assume is par for the course for a particular illness or injury might be incredibly disheartening to the patient who's experiencing it.

This happened to one of my friends when he had minor surgery for a heart problem. He was healing nicely, but then he took a long motorcycle ride, and the constant vibration of the bike combined with the force needed to steer it was a bit too much too soon. Within a couple of days, he had swelling in his left arm and chest and some angry bruising besides.

My friend called his doctor, who didn't seem particularly concerned. His instructions were to just be careful and wait for the swelling and bruising to subside. The doctor didn't think that what happened was a big deal because, to him, it was a fairly typical setback that would easily be overcome with rest and avoiding reinjury. My friend, however, was not so easily appeased. Already feeling anxious because of his newly diagnosed heart problem, he felt intense worry about this additional setback. But it was a normal part of the healing process.

This is why it's so important to me to address the issue of setbacks and plateaus in this book. It can be terribly discouraging to be making progress toward healing, only to have something stand in your way. But by recognizing this as the normal course of recovery, you can maintain your motivation and stay on track, physically and emotionally.

Recognizing Setbacks

We expect setbacks in most areas of life. Consider what baseball commissioner Francis Vincent said in a speech to university students: "Baseball teaches us, or has taught most of us, how to deal with failure. We learn at a very young age that failure is the norm in baseball and, precisely because we have failed, we hold in high regard those who fail less often—those who hit safely in one out of three chances and become star players."

Striking out in baseball and in other areas of life doesn't automatically mean failure in the end. The classic example is Babe Ruth, the original home run king, who held the record for the most strikeouts. But he isn't the only one who achieved success despite, or perhaps because of, failure.

- Henry Ford neglected to put a reverse gear in his first car. He failed and went broke five times before finally succeeding.

- Author Richard Hooker had his novel *MASH* rejected 21 times before he found a publisher. The book became a blockbuster movie and a highly successful television series.

- The mother of Arthur Wellesley, the first Duke of Ellington, considered her son a dunce. While a student at Eton College, he was called dull, idle, and slow. At age 46, he defeated Napoleon, the greatest general living—except, of course, for Wellington.

- An editor of the *Atlantic Monthly* rejected the work of an aspiring young writer named Robert Frost. In a curt note, the editor wrote: "Our magazine has no room for your vigorous verse."

Life may be filled with setbacks and plateaus, but, as the experiences of these gentlemen reveal, the final outcome is not necessarily determined by impediments to the process. Of course, doctors and patients should do what they can to avoid or at least limit physical setbacks. But this isn't always possible, which is why it's helpful to anticipate and acknowledge them as a normal part of the healing process.

One of my colleagues, Carolyn Kaelin, MD, is a surgical oncologist. She was well aware of the setbacks that routinely occur among patients undergoing treatment for breast cancer. Still, it didn't entirely prepare her for the setbacks that awaited her when she received her own diagnosis. In her book called *Living Through Breast Cancer*—an excellent resource for women with the disease—Dr. Kaelin describes her experience. At age 42, she was training for a cycling cancer fund-raiser when she noticed what she says was "the tiniest, most subtle area of skin pulling inward on my right breast." She opted for breast-conserving surgery (a lumpectomy rather than a mastectomy), hoping that all of the cancer cells would be removed. They weren't. She underwent a second lumpectomy, but still cancer cells were left behind. A third lumpectomy failed as well. Finally, with no other viable options, she underwent a mastectomy followed by breast reconstructive surgery.

Five surgeries after her initial diagnosis, Dr. Kaelin could move forward with the rest of her treatment and her recovery from breast cancer. She most certainly had to deal with a lot of physical pain and emotional heartache along the way, but these setbacks did not affect her prognosis. They just made her journey through the Healing Zone more challenging.

Why Setbacks Occur

I once asked sport psychologist Jim Taylor, PhD, about dealing with setbacks, and he offered some interesting insights. According to Dr. Taylor, the types of setbacks that occur with healing fall into two categories: physical and psychological. The physical setbacks are part of the healing process and aren't entirely avoidable. The psychological setbacks are avoidable if people understand their injuries or illnesses and have realistic expectations for recovery. "The psychological setbacks are not inevitable," he said. "But when they occur, they make the physical setbacks worse."

Setbacks may occur for a variety of reasons. Sometimes they happen because people try to rush the healing process by becoming too active too soon. I see this in my patients who ignore what I call the "voice of the body."

One young man was mending from back surgery. He went on a walk with his girlfriend but about halfway through started having pain in his back. Instead of staying where he was and asking his girlfriend to fetch the car, he ignored the pain and finished the walk. A few hours later, he was in excruciating agony. His girlfriend called me in tears, asking what could be done. I asked her to put him on the phone, and I reassured him that it probably would be just a minor setback, easily overcome in a few days with rest and medication. I also told him that pushing himself physically without regard for his pain level was not a good idea so early in the healing process.

I urged him to pay close attention to the voice of his body and let that voice help dictate what he was safely able to do.

Other times setbacks occur as a complication of treatment, as was the case with my friend who had the heart problem. Did he make a mistake in trying to ride his motorcycle too soon? Well, yes and no. In retrospect, he probably should have waited a bit longer, though it's impossible for anyone to predict exactly when it's okay to return to specific activities. Even experienced doctors can only estimate how quickly recovery is progressing and when it is safe to resume one's usual routine. While it's good to be careful, being overly cautious and afraid to do what you enjoy can lead to problems associated with inactivity, including physical deconditioning and emotional frustration or even depression. As Sophia Loren once said, "Mistakes are part of the dues one pays for a full life."

Sometimes setbacks happen because a patient opted for one kind of treatment over another or because a better treatment wasn't recommended or available at the time. This is what happened to Karen Horowitz, a patient of mine whom you may remember from Chapter 11. Karen is a three-time breast cancer survivor. The first time, the cancer was caught at a very early stage due to an irregularity on a routine mammogram. Karen underwent a lumpectomy without any other treatment. Six months later, the cancer returned. Karen underwent another lumpectomy without any other treatment. She did well until her 5-year follow-up, when the cancer had returned yet again. This time she underwent a mastectomy, chemotherapy, and radiation treatment. In Karen's case, the treatment guidelines changed since her initial diagnosis. She says that if she were to get the same early-stage diagnosis today, she would opt for more aggressive treatment than just a lumpectomy.

Acknowledging Plateaus

As with setbacks, it's common and quite normal for people to experience plateaus in the healing process, where they neither progress nor regress. Plateaus can occur for the same reasons as setbacks, and they can be overcome in a similar fashion.

At one point in my recovery from cancer and its treatment, I found myself facing a healing plateau. I knew that my strength and endurance weren't optimal, and I wanted some expert guidance to figure out what to do next. I decided to consult a highly skilled personal trainer, who put me through some fitness tests, identified and evaluated my deficits, and gave me a structured, individualized exercise program to target the areas where I still was weak. This worked fabulously, and soon after I met with him, I began to make progress again.

A different sort of healing plateau can develop for people who require continued medical treatment at certain intervals through the healing process. For example, David Eustace—the little boy whose legs were crushed by an out-of-control car—underwent multiple surgeries and other procedures during the time that he was in the Healing Zone. The same is true for Chris Penrod, who suffered severe burns over 90 percent of his body in a fire at his workplace. His recovery involved many surgical procedures, including numerous skin grafts. Chris's Remarkable Recovery story is at the end of this chapter.

No matter what sort of healing plateau you might face, always remind yourself that it's just part of the process. Nancy Davis, a woman with multiple sclerosis who has become an advocate for others with the condition, offers this bit of wisdom: "There is no failure, only feedback." It's a healthy perspective that can assist you not only in continuing your journey through the Healing Zone but also in reevaluating your goals. If you find yourself on a bumpy path with lots of roadblocks, change directions to find a smoother ride.

How to Overcome Physical Setbacks and Plateaus

To cope with and even overcome setbacks and plateaus on the path to Super Healing, you do have several tools and techniques at your disposal. Before we discuss them, I want to reiterate that the first and most important step in addressing setbacks and plateaus is to simply acknowledge their existence as part and parcel of the healing process. Most likely you still can heal well despite them.

While I can offer some general guidance on navigating setbacks and plateaus, the more educated you are about your particular condition, the better you will be able to avoid them or deal with them if they do occur. You also want to know what might lie ahead, so you can prepare for it as much as possible. Your best resource is your medical doctor—your conductor for your journey through the Healing Zone. He or she can answer your questions and alleviate any uncertainty.

As you'll remember, my friend with the heart problem called his physician about the swelling and bruising he was experiencing. His doctor explained that this complication can happen in the first few weeks after the particular procedure he had undergone. The doctor reassured him that the swelling would resolve and likely wouldn't happen again.

When I talked with my friend about this setback, I told him that what happened was a normal part of the healing process and that he should believe his doctor, who is well respected and very experienced, having performed hundreds if not thousands of the same procedure. His reassurance was genuine and accurate. Other health care professionals also can be extremely helpful in this way.

Friends and family, while well meaning, usually are not good sources of medical advice—unless they have extensive training and expertise in your particular condition. Elizabeth Edwards, who found out she had breast cancer during her husband's vice presidential campaign in 2004, learned this during the first week after her diagnosis. In her book *Saving Graces*, she describes a phone conversation with Teresa Heinz in which Heinz said, "There are plenty of good doctors . . . Just don't use . . . " The doctor she named happened to be one that Edwards was seeing.

In her book, Edwards writes, "There were real valleys in this process, and sometimes the valleys are precipitated by little pieces of misinformation from which no one can really protect you. And on that first weekend, Teresa's warning—which we concluded was wrong—sent me into a real valley." In my experience, even the kindest friends can cause tremendous anxiety when they offer inaccurate if well-intentioned medical advice. Consult your health care team instead.

Karen Horowitz, the three-time breast cancer survivor and now cancer advocate, shares this insight.

> I always tell people with a new cancer diagnosis to take a step back and think about what they want to do. Don't get rushed or pushed into any decision. I know too many people who were so afraid that they did things very fast, and they didn't always find the right doctors and have the best treatment. So I tell people to sort of take that step back, look at what your options are, talk to people, get input, and don't do anything until you feel that you're making the best decision for you, and not for anybody else. A lot of people have said, "My husband thinks, my friends think . . . " And I tell them, "No, this is about you."

With all this in mind, here are some suggestions to help you move beyond physical setbacks and plateaus.

Make an appointment with your doctor to discuss what is happening. Be clear about your symptoms and why you are concerned. Maybe you need a different medical treatment than you've been getting. Or perhaps your doctor will offer reassurance that you just need to wait a bit longer for this phase of healing to proceed.

Assess why you aren't meeting your goals. Are they too hard, or will they simply take longer to achieve than you anticipated? Have you spent enough time trying to accomplish them? If not, don't be discouraged. It's perfectly understandable that with everything else going on, you may not have been able to focus your time and energy on tackling certain goals. Simply acknowledge this and recommit yourself to working toward them.

Shift your focus to the parts of your body that are working well. In the previous chapter, I suggested strengthening regions of your body that are already strong. This can instill confidence and help facilitate whole-body healing.

Be patient and persevere. Overcoming setbacks and plateaus takes time. If you've done everything you can to move forward and it just isn't happening, then relax and let time be on your side. Of course, this is easier said than done. It might help to remember that sometimes healing takes place in such small increments that though you can't see or feel your progress, it's occurring.

How to Avoid Psychological Setbacks

Often you can avoid psychological setbacks or at least limit the damage they can cause. I tend to think of psychological setbacks as falling into two distinct categories. The first consists of situations in which something actually happening to you is causing an emotional response. In the second category are situations that I call ambushes, which are created by the people around you and don't involve you personally.

Let's start with the ambushes, because they are relatively easy to deal with once you can recognize them. By my definition, an ambush has the following two characteristics.

1. It is some kind of news that causes your mood to plummet.
2. It has nothing to do with your particular health situation.

Ambushes happen to people in the Healing Zone all the time for a variety of reasons. You can detect them because they come without warning and suddenly change how you feel. A good example of an ambush is what happened to Elizabeth Edwards when she was talking to Teresa Heinz. Well-meaning friends can inadvertently ambush someone who's in the Healing Zone.

I can't begin to count how many people have told me their worst-case cancer stories. Though I try to be polite, for my own sanity's sake, I usually try to cut off such conversations before they get too far along. If my children are present, I tend to be a bit more curt, as they, too, are at risk for being ambushed.

Whenever people unintentionally ambush me, I tell myself (and my children, if they are witnesses) that they are genuinely well-meaning and may be sharing something that is painful for me because they are suffering themselves. Nevertheless, it's good to recognize that what these people say is an ambush and put it into proper perspective. For instance, if someone tells me a worst-case cancer story, I remind myself that they are not talking about me and that my situation is in no way connected to whatever information they are sharing.

The media is another potential source of ambushes. While sometimes news reports offer information about promising new treatments, they too often focus on tragic stories that can upset people who are in the Healing Zone. Back in Chapter 10, I mentioned the phrase "If it bleeds, it leads." It's a fairly accurate description of today's news coverage, and it can lead to many unnecessary ambushes while you are in the Healing Zone. Recognize these ambushes for what they are. If you find that your mood is plummeting, ask yourself whether the information truly is applicable to you and your situation.

The second category of psychological setbacks is specific to your medical condition. One of the best ways to deal with these setbacks is to try to anticipate what might happen so you can prepare for it. I don't mean you should worry about every possible side effect from a medication or a procedure, but do have realistic expectations about how long you will need to heal and what might happen during this time.

When I give talks to people recovering from cancer treatment, invariably I discover that many of them don't have a good sense of the duration of the recovery period after chemotherapy, radiation, or other therapies. For the majority of cancer patients, this period is measured in months or years rather than weeks. Yet people routinely come up to me and say, "It's been 6 weeks, and I still feel terrible." Reassuring them that they will feel better, but it's going to take much longer than 6 weeks, helps them put their situations in the proper perspective and not become overly discouraged.

For my friend—and perhaps for you, too—being aware of possible setbacks and getting reassurance from his doctor didn't completely alleviate his concerns. It's extremely difficult to suffer a setback in the midst of healing. All of us just want to get better as quickly as possible.

Setbacks are beyond annoying; they are discouraging, and they can be quite devastating. My friend did what I suggest to others, which is to talk with people whom you trust. His wife was tremendously supportive, regularly reminding him of his doctor's words. He also talked with me, and I was able to confirm for him that his physician likely was correct in assessing his situation.

Some people will seek out second or third opinions from doctors, which is fine. Whenever a patient tells me that she wants another opinion, I embrace her decision and ask her to share with me what the other doctor says. In most cases, the doctor will recommend the same things that I did. But sometimes he or she thinks of things that I didn't or has relevant experience that I don't. It isn't unusual for me to refer my patients to other doctors, even within my own specialty. I always tell my patients that my main objective is to help them heal, and sometimes it means listening to what other experts have to say.

In summary, here's what you can do to avoid psychological setbacks or deal with them when they arise.

Recognize an ambush when it happens. Realize that it has nothing to do with you or your situation, and dismiss it without another thought.

Talk with your doctor about anything that pertains to setbacks or plateaus you are experiencing. He or she will be able to help troubleshoot your situation so you can move forward again. Short of that, at least he or she can confirm that the situation is normal and will resolve eventually.

Consider getting a second or third opinion. Every doctor should welcome the input of an esteemed colleague. This might be incredibly helpful to you from a medical perspective, or it can provide you with much-needed reassurance from a psychological perspective.

Share your feelings with someone you trust. Having a family member or friend to talk with is a great way to diminish worry and angst. Just saying something out loud often lessens the emotional burden you are carrying.

Look at How Far You've Come

As I mentioned in the previous chapter, it's very helpful to review your goals and evaluate whether they are realistic and how best to go about achieving them. Goals that are unrealistic can make you feel like a failure when in fact you may be healing quite well.

It isn't always easy to know what a realistic goal is, however. The brilliant writer Alice Walker offers us excellent advice in this regard when she tells us to "plan, but don't plan as if it will all happen as you planned it." If you have experienced a setback or a healing plateau, review your goals and decide whether they need to be adjusted a bit.

Dr. Taylor, the sports psychologist, shares a terrific piece of advice that he offers to competitive athletes who sustain serious injuries. He counsels them to think about "the here and now, and then the distance." He tells them not to focus on the middle of the journey, since that often is the most unpredictable part of recovery. In other words, he is suggesting that you concentrate on what you need to do today to achieve your goals and then on how you will feel when you have completed the mending process. As Dr. Taylor says, "Maintaining a long-term perspective is important. No one rehab session will predict your recovery."

For most people, traveling through the Healing Zone takes more time than they'd like. You can alleviate the burden of the journey just by recognizing and even celebrating the progress you've made. Look back to where you started and see how far you've come. If you achieve one of your goals, mark it with a celebration. This can be something simple, such as buying yourself an inexpensive beaded bracelet as a visual reminder of what you've accomplished. Or do something special you've been wanting to do—see a movie, eat at a favorite restaurant, take a walk in the park. It really doesn't matter how you choose to celebrate. Just the act of commemorating your progress will help you through your journey.

Finally, above all else, remember that you are extraordinarily resilient. You have many untapped resources that you may need to tap in your quest to Super Heal.

REMARKABLE RECOVERY

Chris Penrod

In January 1998, I was in a flash fire. I was 29 years old at the time. I suffered burns to 90 percent of my body, with 70 percent being third-degree, the most serious type.

I was working as a mechanic in one room, and there were guys working with a torch near a gas can in another room. When I walked into the room they were in, a spark hit the gas can and the fumes blew up. There were two of us who were injured bad. The other guys just had burns on their hands, trying to put us out.

I remember everything. I walked by where they were working, I reached in the toolbox, something popped, and I was covered in flames. I ran out the door and tried to do the stop, drop, and roll, but it didn't work. So I got up and started running. Then I heard a voice call me back, someone that had a hose. I ran to him and he put me out.

I didn't know how bad I was burned. I must have been in shock because I just said, "All I need is another uniform." I never saw my body. But they said, "No, no. You've got to wait for the ambulance." I said, "No, I can just change." Then the ambulance showed up, and they started pulling the bed out. I said, "No. I can walk in." I walked in, sat down, and that's when the pain hit.

They were pouring water on me all the way to the hospital. They got me on the table. They were putting tubes in me, and I was screaming. The doctor just grabbed my hand and said everything was going to be all right. And then I basically woke out of an induced coma 2 months later.

The doctors said I was in bad shape, but I didn't understand until like a year later that I almost died a few times in there. My family came to visit me every day, though I didn't know it. When it first happened, they called all my family and everybody came. I guess the doctors told them to say good-bye because they didn't think I was going to make it.

Once I woke up, I just wanted to get better and get out of there. So I did everything I had to do—walk, move my hands. I had to learn to walk again, because I guess you forget while you're in that induced coma. I started walking around, and I knew I was going to get better. But I didn't know how good I was going to get. I decided that I was going to try to be as good as I could get with the help of the doctors and therapy.

The first surgery I had was a big one. My arm was almost welded to my side, so they wanted to release the arm by making cuts. You could see the releases. They wanted to make so many cuts, so they said I'd have to be in the hospital for a week. It took a whole week, and they did a lot of work. They took a skin graft about an inch and a half, 2 inches wide from underneath my armpit all the way down to my knee, to replace the skin that they were cutting and to make my arm straighter and have more flexibility. I have had a lot of other surgeries, too.

I'm at the point now where I can pick and choose when I want my next surgeries. They said I could fix my thumbs, my fingers. Whatever's wrong now, they can make it better, but they can't fix it totally. I've been putting it off for the last couple of years. You get to a point where you have had enough. Leave me alone. I'm doing well, I can dress myself, and I can drive a car. But this won't last forever. I know that my skin will start to tighten up more and I won't be feeling as well. Eventually I'm going to do it. I just want to have a couple of years without going through all that, and kind of living a normal life.

For a long time I was angry about the fact that my accident could have been prevented. I thought about the guys who started the fire, and I thought that might have been me doing that, and someone else walking in the room. I put myself in their position. They have to live with the fact that they burned someone as bad as they did me. They have to live with that. So forgiveness was a big thing in my recovery. I talked to the guy who was doing the torching, and I forgave him. I mean, why should he live like that? It could have been anybody.

I can't remember being normal, whatever normal is. It's like this accident happened, and I'm here, and this is the way my life is now. I can't remember it being any different. It took a long time to get to this point, but I'm here. I can't remember not having burnt skin. I look at pictures of me when I was younger and it's like, wow, what would it be like not to have this? But I do. I have to deal with it.

About a year after my injury, I started going back to the burn unit to talk to other patients. Afterward, I would cry all the way home. It was good, though. It was good to talk to people.

Chapter 15

Continue the Healing Journey

If you are reading this chapter, then you've got what it takes to Super Heal—namely, knowledge, patience, and perseverance. I've covered a lot of territory in this book, and you've stuck with it. Not everyone would.

I remember an encounter with one woefully impatient man—not a patient but a fellow passenger on an airplane. I had just settled into my seat when I heard a commotion a couple of rows behind me. Apparently, a very young woman was taking a long time to get settled in. She was listening to her iPod and didn't realize this man was waiting behind her. Other passengers saw his frustration and heard him make some disparaging remarks. Finally fed up with the young woman, he decided to teach her a lesson by deliberately hitting her with his carry-on bag (or so the eyewitnesses reported).

This man—a slightly overweight, middle-aged businessman—vehemently denied striking the young woman on purpose. But according to the flight attendant, the captain insisted that the man disembark. He argued and then demanded to talk with the captain personally. After about 10 minutes, the man returned to his seat and collected his belongings, and the flight attendant escorted him off the plane. We then departed for our destination, minus one passenger.

Whether you are on a real journey or a metaphorical healing journey, it takes time, and rushing may lead to unintended—and possibly negative—consequences. All of us would like to be at our desired destinations instantaneously, but no journey works that way.

The man on the plane needed to learn patience and respect. These qualities go a long way in supporting physical recovery as well—patience for the time you need to heal and respect for your body as it mends. I know this may be easier said than done, but consider the alternative. For the man on the plane, his journey no doubt took far longer to complete, perhaps with unanticipated obstacles to navigate (it was rumored that he was taken into custody by airport security personnel). For the person who needs to heal, impatience can lead to setbacks, which can delay or even change the ultimate outcome.

Of course, this might seem to run counter to the realities of modern life, which moves at an increasingly fast pace and demands nearly instant gratification. My son, a teenage musician, will finish jazz band practice after school and then call me on his cell phone for a ride home. Ten minutes later, he is getting into the front seat of the car and asking, "Mom, what took you so long?" My son is a wonderful young man who is patient by nature. But at this time of day, he is tired and hungry, and he has hours of homework in front of him. For him, waiting 10 minutes seems like a long time.

All of my children and their friends, as well as most adults, have an expectation of speed. But this expectation doesn't usually fit in the context of healing. As my young saxophonist knows, musicians use the phrase *tempo giusto,* which means "the right speed." In great music, as in healing, it is the right speed that matters.

Take the Time to Heal Optimally

For many people with serious illnesses or injuries, the 1-year time frame of the Super Healing Plan is ideal. Others, though, need more time than that.

At a talk that I was giving to cancer survivors, I met a woman who said she had been diagnosed with cancer in the 1970s. (This happened in 2006.) At the time, she was told she had less than 6 months to live. This woman opted for very aggressive treatment that lasted for more than 4 years and included 28 surgeries or other procedures (e.g., bone marrow transplantation). Her husband tried valiantly to keep up her spirits during her treatment; he hung a sign over the door to their home that read something like "If you are going to cry, please leave! We need encouragement and hope." He also went around the house and posted Bible verses in every cabinet, so when she opened a door, the verse was the first thing she saw. Fortunately, she survived, but hers was an especially harrowing experience. Not surprisingly, she needed several years to heal as well as possible.

After my cancer treatment, it took me about 2 years to reach roughly 90 percent of my healing capacity. Basically, I did the Super Healing Plan twice. After the first year, when I realized I still had a ways to go, I just started again and set new goals. This is easy to do, especially if you already have done it once.

Even if you have a chronic medical condition, you need time to optimize your physical health. You can use 12 months as your first marker, and then decide whether to repeat the plan. The beauty of the Super Healing Plan is that while it covers a finite period, it helps you adopt health habits that I hope will stay with you for life.

Many people, even my close friends, were surprised by how long I needed to really begin feeling like myself again. They wanted me to feel better right away. Though I wished for that, too, it just wasn't possible.

I rarely opened up to others about how much I was struggling during this time, but during a conversation with one of my friends, I mentioned how hard the healing journey really was. She was shocked because she thought I was all better. She said, "But you walk around with a smile on your face. I had no idea you were still healing!"

I realized then that I had simply assumed that those around me would know that I hadn't fully recovered and that my healing journey was taking many months. I also realized that by not saying anything to my friend, she had mistakenly interpreted the fact that I was smiling and pleasant as a sign that I felt really good physically. I remember thinking to myself, "Wow, I faked out one of my closest friends!" But I didn't mean to. I assumed some things, and she assumed some things, and neither of us really knew what the other was thinking.

I've learned that this is a pretty common scenario. People tend to look better than they feel, and if they don't specifically tell their loved ones what is going on, then those to whom they are closest assume that they feel better than they do. Another way to think of this is that people tend to heal more quickly on the outside than they do on the inside. It simply takes longer for all of the different organs and tissues inside our bodies to heal well.

This occurred to me one day as a woman who is a cancer survivor and her best friend approached me at a talk I was giving. The woman said, "My best friend knows that I still don't feel well, but my husband doesn't want to believe that I still don't feel well." By asking a couple of questions about her husband, I found out that, in general, he was a very kind and loving man. I suspected that two things may have created the misunderstanding between them. First, the wife may have assumed that her husband understood more than he did about how she was physically feeling. Just because her friend understood, it didn't mean that her husband did not need more explanation. Second, as often happens, those who love us most want so much for us to feel better that they may somewhat deceive themselves into believing it's true.

Since it took me about 2 years to heal optimally, the last thing I wanted to do was confide in every person I met about the fact that I still was mending. Instead, I learned to be honest and talk with the people closest to me at regular intervals. Of course, incessant complaining doesn't help anyone. While it's a good idea to let your loved ones know how you feel, it's also best to do this just on occasion so they—and you—don't feel the constant burden of the healing journey.

When I say that I felt about 90 percent better after 2 years, I am just estimating. But it took me about that long to be close to feeling as good physically as I was going to ever feel again. It wasn't quite as good as I would have felt if I had never had cancer or cancer treatment, but it was much, much better than I had felt at the end of my chemotherapy regimen. I say "90 percent" because almost everyone who travels through the Healing Zone—including me—has areas that they can continue to work on to physically improve their health.

What You Need to Super Heal

For me to say that I was patient throughout my time in the Healing Zone would not be accurate. I am not naturally inclined to be patient. But one thing that helped me to relax and accept what often seemed to be the very slow pace of physical healing was the knowledge that I was doing what I could to provide my body with what it needed to recover optimally. Basically, I was doing everything that I could to heal.

This isn't to say I did everything exactly right. I didn't. In fact, it would be practically impossible over the course of a year or more. There were days when I ate too much junk food and days when I moped instead of going out to exercise. There were many nights—especially in the beginning—when no matter what I did, I couldn't sleep a solid 8 hours.

Still, I was able to Super Heal, because what it really means to Super Heal is to:

- Focus on the primary Super Healing Synergy that involves the three most important healing parameters: therapeutic exercise to build strength and endurance, food to nourish and promote healing, and proper rest to encourage optimal immune function and recovery.

- Consider the other things that may affect your ability to mend. These include alleviating pain, using mind-body techniques, treating or preventing prolonged mood problems such as depression, recognizing the importance of love and connections, and tapping into spirituality.

- Set specific goals that encompass these important healing concepts and encourage you to progress as quickly as possible.

- Expect some setbacks and don't allow them to derail your journey, either physically or emotionally.

- Do the best you can. Keep in mind that your body wants to heal and that any help you give it is extremely valuable.

While you are in the Healing Zone, the things outlined in this book will help you to heal. As you emerge from the Healing Zone, these same things will help you remain as strong and healthy as possible. I have found that people who are facing serious illness or injury often are highly motivated. They can use this motivation not only to recover but also to create new health habits. The good news is that after the Super Healing Plan ends, you won't have any extra work ahead of you to create these great new habits. You just need to keep on doing what you've been doing all along.

I often share the story of my mother-in-law, who was struck down by a stroke when she was in her early forties. With eight children to raise, she worked extremely hard to heal. Though her recovery took time, she focused on the most important aspects of healing. These became lifetime habits for her. Today she is in her seventies, and she is quite remarkable in her vigor and good health. There is no doubt that her stroke propelled her to make some changes that not only facilitated her recovery but also had a dramatic impact on her health throughout her life.

Some people might see this as a gift that comes out of a serious illness. I have a hard time seeing any illness as a gift, but I do think that every experience—whether it's good or bad—opens the door to change. Facing serious illness allows us to stop and reflect in a way that might not otherwise be possible. Out of this can come wonderful opportunities to choose a new direction or path you might not have previously considered taking.

Finding Your Middle Ground

As I have mentioned throughout this book, Super Healing is about optimal recovery from serious illness or injury. It is not about curing chronic conditions, nor is it about healing perfectly with no physical or emotional scars or limitations. There are so many occasions in my practice when I see a patient who's really struggling and think, "If I had a magic wand, I would instantly cure this person." But there are no magic wands in medicine. The tools of our trade are science and compassion. Though I often wish for a little sorcery to help my patients feel better, it simply isn't possible.

I have seen literally thousands of people travel through the Healing Zone, and no journey was exactly the same as any other. Most of the people I shepherd through recovery, whether they have a new illness or injury or a chronic one, come to accept whatever limitations they have. It doesn't mean that they are happy about these limitations; it just means that they are able to move beyond them and lead meaningful lives.

While most individuals strike a balance between working hard toward their recovery and accepting their losses, I've seen two groups of people who end up with more disability than they need to live with. In the first group are those who are overly accepting of their limitations. These folks assume that as they age, they'll become very decrepit, and they're better off just going along with it rather than fighting it. This mind-set is not based in science, which shows that as we get older, we can make tremendous gains in our physical endurance, strength, mobility, and so on just by utilizing the sort of tools and techniques that I offer in the Super Healing Plan. The second group consists of people who are unwilling to accept any limitations. They want to be just as they were before, and if this isn't possible, they simply give up.

Healing optimally usually involves some compromise. You may need to settle for less than you want in order to achieve the best possible outcome. These are lessons that we have had to learn throughout our lives, though a few people will always opt out if they can't get exactly what they want.

This reminds me of a story that my daughter told me about her schoolyard playmates. One child in particular tries to control all of the games. This little girl appoints herself as the leader and will select my daughter and another child to play with. Then, when a fourth girl asks to play, the self-appointed leader will promptly tell her, "This game can only be played with three kids." My daughter doesn't like this, so she tells the fourth child, "Of course you can play, and we'll take turns or make teams." Whereupon the leader—who is desperately trying to maintain control—replies with, "Okay, then I'm not going to play."

These are innocent children who have much to learn about compromise, leadership, and friendship, and the playground is a place where they can hone skills that will help them later in life. There is no doubt that compromise is essential on the journey through the Healing Zone. Employing this child's technique of opting out when she doesn't get exactly what she wants is not especially useful when you're trying to recover optimally.

Your Final Destination

The stories that the media adores are those featuring people who face tremendous adversity, then go on to Super Heal with seemingly no lasting effects. These people are hailed as heroes who inspire us with their monumental achievements.

One of my favorite media heroes is Lance Armstrong, who was diagnosed with testicular cancer that had spread to his brain. Lance traveled through the Healing Zone and came out the other side to become a cycling legend with seven Tour de France victories. He also has done incredible work on behalf of the cancer community. In his case, the media's (mostly) positive portrayal of him is hard-won and well deserved.

But what happens when the end result isn't a series of Tour de France victories? What happens to guys like Joe Theismann, who don't heal completely?

As you may recall, Theismann—a former Washington Redskins quarterback—was voted the National Football League's Most Valuable Player in 1983. His phenomenal 12-year professional football career came to an abrupt halt on a Monday night in 1985, when New York Giants defensive lineman Lawrence Taylor tackled him. In an interview published in the book *Rising to the Challenge*, Theismann describes what happened.

> I handed the ball to John Riggins, he turned around and pitched it back to me as he ran toward the line of scrimmage. When I caught it, I looked downfield. I was supposed to throw a deep post-pattern to one of my wide receivers, but the safety wasn't fooled. So I was looking for the secondary receiver and I couldn't quite locate the tight end who was supposed to be on the right side. And then I felt some pressure coming from my left side. So I thought I'd step up into the pocket for safety. And as it turns out, Lawrence Taylor grabbed my left shoulder. I was standing rigid in the pocket with my feet firmly planted, and as he swung around, his thigh caught my right leg between my ankle and my knee. [It] just snapped my leg like a toothpick. I remember hearing a "pow, pow." It sounded like two muzzled gunshots. It was actually my leg breaking!

Though injuries often end athletic careers, Theismann and his teammates and coaches all hoped that he would fully recover. At first it looked like he would. Theismann describes his journey through the Healing Zone.

> When I first started therapy, and got out of the cast, I was pleased by the amount of progress I was making. I did everything the doctors and trainers prescribed for me. I would take it to the max, as far as the therapy would go. I would not only work on my leg but work on the rest of my body so that when my leg was healed every part of me would be in good shape. The early part of recovery was really encouraging because I could see large amounts of improvement.
>
> Then after about six or seven months, the improvements started decreasing. The increments were much smaller, still fairly noticeable, but much smaller. . . . I started to try and do football-type movements. . . . Then all of a sudden, I realized I had lost about 20 percent strength in my right leg. No matter how hard I

worked, no matter what I did, I was still unable to get back to the strength that I had.

While Theismann remains a tremendous athlete, he wasn't able to resume playing professional football. He says, "Emotionally, for me, I think the toughest times came after leaving the game. While I was still training, while I was still fighting through it, I'd get so frustrated. I'd get so frustrated at times when I was training. I'd cry. And throw things. I was not a very pleasant person to be around because, hell, I wanted to be well. I wanted to play."

I have no doubt that Theismann did Super Heal. But as he learned on his journey through the Healing Zone, as you work to physically recover, you may encounter health issues that ultimately determine your final destination. Knowing what to accept and what not to so often is very difficult to define. Talk with your doctors about your expectations and theirs. Keep in mind that many patients exceed their doctors' expectations through hard work and determination.

Interestingly, Theismann—who has gone on to do many wonderful things with his life, including motivational speaking—has this philosophy: "Most people look at what happened to me as a tragedy in sports. I look at it as a blessing for a man."

Make the Commitment

Once you commit yourself to a given task, things tend to fall into place in a manner you couldn't have predicted. It is as if the stars align and work in your favor. In a passage from the book *The Scottish Himalayan Expedition*, W. H. Murray explains how commitment works.

> Until one is committed, there is hesitancy. . . . The moment one definitely commits oneself, then Providence moves, too. All sorts of things occur to help one that would never otherwise have occurred. A whole stream of events raising in one's favor . . . unforeseen incidents and meetings and material assistance which no man could have dreamed could have come his way.

I encourage you to commit yourself to healing as optimally as you can. If you are reading this book, chances are you already are in the Healing Zone. Make your journey as safe as possible. Work hard and diligently to ensure that your final destination is the best one for you. Know that there will be bumps in the road; accept them, correct your course as needed, and continue your journey. As my doctor friend who aspires to publish a book said, "Just keep moving the chain."

This is exactly what one of my patients, a polio survivor who needed back surgery, did during his postoperative recovery. Though the surgery went well, he spent the next few months in the Healing Zone. As he was nearing the end of his journey, he asked me what he could do for me, since I had helped him so much with his rehabilitation. My first instinct was to say "nothing," but then I decided that I really did want something. I wanted to know that now that he felt better, he would pursue the travel he had been longing to do. So I said, "Every time you go somewhere, send me a magnet with the name of the city you are in." For years he has been doing this, and now my refrigerator is covered with magnets from the places this lovely man has been.

As you finish your metaphorical healing journey, plan to take a real trip to somewhere special. Then send me an e-mail (via my Web site, www.superhealing.net) from wherever you are. I'd love to hear from you!

Appendix A

The Super Healing Shortcut Plan

At the start of this book, I mentioned that regardless of whether you decide to follow the Super Healing Plan by writing out your goals and working to achieve them, simply reading this information is a big step in the direction of recovery. Educating yourself and gaining knowledge about physical healing surely will help you to heal.

That said, there are many reasons that certain readers won't be able to follow through with the entire plan. Some are simply too sick; some may lack the motivation because they are overwhelmed by other things in their lives; and some simply may not have the inclination to follow a "plan." For these people—and, perhaps, for you—I have developed the Super Healing Shortcut Plan.

Generally, I'm pretty good about following a plan. I like structure, and I love results. But I once had the opportunity to read a terrific book about how to cultivate creativity in yourself. There isn't a lot of room for creativity in conventional medicine, and I was yearning to have more of it in my life. While the author offered a specific plan and plenty of encouragement, I simply didn't have the time to do what she suggested without wreaking havoc in the lives of my husband, children, and patients. Nevertheless, I did adopt some of her suggestions, and I found them to be really helpful.

For me, healing well was a necessity, while fostering creativity was more of a luxury (especially since my livelihood didn't depend on it). Thus, when it came to healing, I did what we talked about in Chapter 4: I made time to heal. This was my priority, and I knew that regaining optimal physical health would be a gift to me as well as to my loved ones.

Of course, I wouldn't have written the Super Healing Plan if I didn't think it was the best way to help you recover optimally. But if you aren't able to start or complete the plan, you can take a shortcut that will enable you to begin tackling the three most important elements of Super Healing—engaging in therapeutic exercise, eating nourishing foods, and obtaining proper rest.

The Super Healing Shortcut Plan doesn't require you to write down anything, and it takes only minimal effort—with the potential outcome being a big boost in your ability to heal. So while I hope that you'll become fully engaged in the Super Healing Plan, if you don't feel up to it now, then try the Super Healing Shortcut Plan. Here's what to do:

1. Count your steps using a pedometer. This will give you an idea of how active you are on a daily basis. It's easy, and it's a lot of fun. My patients tell me that it really helps them get on the path to Super Healing. Occasionally I'll bump into my patients while I'm out and about with my husband or kids. Invariably, they'll lift up their shirts just enough for me to see the pedometers attached to the top of their pants and say, "Look, Dr. Silver, I'm tracking my steps!"

Begin by keeping track of how many steps a day (on average) you are taking. Then gradually increase untill you are up to 10,000 steps per day—the number recommended by the American College of Sports Medicine for active, healthy adults. If this isn't realistic for you, based on where you are in the Healing Zone, then simply start monitoring your activity level and talk with your doctor about whether it's reasonable for you to advance to 10,000 steps per day.

I strongly encourage you to use a pedometer. It's so easy that you don't even need to think about it. Just take it off at night and see how active you've been. In case you're curious, approximately 2,000 steps equals 1 mile.

2. Eat five times per day. This won't work for everyone—those with diabetes or gastrointestinal problems should consult their doctors before trying it—but it's okay for most people. By eating five times per day, I mean three small- to medium-size meals, along with two nutritious snacks. It's one way to boost your energy level while avoiding a drop in blood sugar, which can leave you feeling fatigued.

For most people, a diet that's high in lean protein and low in fat—with several servings of fruits and vegetables per day—is ideal. If you need to gain or lose weight, be conscientious about portion size and consult a dietitian about how often you should be eating. Five times per day is a general guideline; you may need the more specific advice that your doctor or a registered dietitian can provide.

3. Sleep at least 8 hours every night. In order to achieve this, most people need to give up daytime naps and follow the rules of good sleep hygiene (beginning on page 114). Medical intervention is often necessary to control pain, alleviate insomnia, or treat other problems that can interrupt sleep, such as hot flashes. If you are not regularly getting 8 hours of sleep per night, or if you don't awaken feeling refreshed (in the Healing Zone, sleep should generally feel restorative), then talk with your doctor about what you are experiencing.

Appendix B

Where to Find Help

Medical Information

American Academy of Physical Medicine and Rehabilitation (AAPM&R)

330 North Wabash Avenue, Suite 2500
Chicago, IL 60611-7617
312-464-9700

www.aapmr.org

The AAPM&R is the premier national medical society for physicians who specialize in physical medicine and rehabilitation. The Web site has sections for membership, the annual assembly, physicians, residents, medical students, and continuing medical education. There is also industry information and a job board.

American Cancer Society (ACS)

1599 Clifton Road NE
Atlanta, GA 30329
800-ACS-2345 (800-227-2345)

www.cancer.org

ACS is a nationwide community-based volunteer health organization with state divisions and more than 3,400 local offices. Its goal is to eliminate cancer as a major health problem by preventing the disease, saving lives, and diminishing suffering through research, education, advocacy, and service. The Web site has sections for patients, families and friends, survivors, donors and volunteers, and professionals.

American Medical Association (AMA)

515 North State Street
Chicago, IL 60610
800-621-8335
312-464-5000

www.ama-assn.org

The AMA, the country's largest physicians' group, develops and promotes standards in medical practice, research, and education. The consumer health information section on the association's Web site has databases on physicians and hospitals that can be searched by medical specialty, as well as information on specific conditions.

National Center for Complementary and Alternative Medicine (NCCAM)

PO Box 7923
Gaithersburg, MD 20898
888-644-6226
866-464-3615 (TTY)

www.nccam.nih.gov

NCCAM explores complementary and alternative healing practices through research, research training and education, outreach, and integration. The Web site offers publications, information for researchers, frequently asked questions, and links to other CAM-related resources. The NCCAM Clearinghouse is the public's source for scientifically based information on CAM and information about NCCAM.

National Institutes of Health (NIH)

9000 Rockville Pike
Bethesda, MD 20892
800 4-CANCER (800-422-6237)
800-332-8615 (TTY)

www.nih.gov

The NIH is a focal point for medical research in the United States. Comprised of 27 institutes and centers, it is an agency of the Public Health Service, a division of the U.S. Department of Health and Human Services. NIH research acquires new knowledge to help prevent, detect, diagnose, and treat disease and disability.

National Library of Medicine (NLM)

8600 Rockville Pike
Bethesda, MD 20894
888-FIND-NLM (888-346-3656)

www.nlm.nih.gov

The NLM collects, organizes, and makes available biomedicine and health care information to medical professionals and offers programs for medical library services in the United States. Both health professionals and the public use its electronic databases extensively throughout the world. Materials are available in multiple languages.

Lance Armstrong Foundation
PO Box 161150
Austin, TX 78716-1150
512-236-8820

www.laf.org

The Lance Armstrong Foundation was founded in 1997 by cancer survivor and champion cyclist Lance Armstrong. The LAF provides practical information and tools that people living with cancer need to survive. LAF's mission is to inspire and empower people with cancer. Visit the Web site to learn more about the foundation's opportunities for education, advocacy, public health, and research programs.

Nutrition

American Dietetic Association (ADA)
120 South Riverside Plaza, Suite 2000
Chicago, IL 60606-6995
800-877-1600

www.eatright.org

The ADA, the world's largest organization of food and nutrition professionals, promotes nutrition, health, and well-being. The Web site has information on diet and nutrition and publications, as well as a registered dietitian locator service, which includes dietitians who specialize in oncology nutrition.

Harvard School of Public Health
Department of Nutrition
665 Huntington Avenue
Boston, MA 02115
617-432-1851

www.hsph.harvard.edu/nutritionsource/

The Nutrition Source, a Web site maintained by the department of nutrition at the Harvard School of Public Health, serves as a resource for the most up-to-date information on diet and nutrition and dispels rumors and fallacies about fad diets.

MyPyramid Tracker

www.mypyramidtracker.gov

The Interactive Healthy Eating Index is an online dietary- and physical-assessment tool developed by the USDA's Center for Nutrition Policy and Promotion. It provides information on diet quality and physical activity status.

International Food Information Council (IFIC) Foundation
1100 Connecticut Avenue NW, Suite 430
Washington, DC 20036
202-296-6540

www.ific.org

IFIC Foundation offers science-based information on food safety and nutrition to health and nutrition professionals, educators, journalists, and others. The IFIC partners with a wide range of professional organizations and academic institutions to develop science-based information for the public.

Meals on Wheels Association of America (MOWAA)
203 South Union Street
Alexandria, VA 22314
703-548-5558

www.mowaa.org

Meals on Wheels is a membership association that offers programs to provide home-delivered and group meals. The organization aims to improve the quality of life of the needy. Some programs may provide other health and social services.

National Heart, Lung, and Blood Institute Health Information Center
Attention: Web Site
PO Box 30105
Bethesda, MD 20824-0105
301-592-8573
240-629-3255 (TTY)
Calculating your body mass index:

www.nhlbisupport.com/bmi

This Web site provides information about body mass index and what constitutes a healthy weight for both men and women. It also provides links to information about controlling food and planning menus.

USDA Food and Nutrition Information Center (FNIC)

National Agricultural Library

10301 Baltimore Avenue, Room 105

Beltsville, MD 20705

301-504-5719

301-504-5414 (for inquiries to dietitians and nutritionists)

www.nal.usda.gov/fnic

The USDA's FNIC is an information center for the National Agricultural Library. FNIC materials and services include dietitians and nutritionists available to answer inquiries, publications on food and nutrition, and resource lists and bibliographies. The FNIC Web site includes information on dietary supplements, food safety, dietary guidelines, food composition facts (including fast food), a list of available publications, and information on popular topics.

United States Food and Drug Administration (FDA)

5600 Fishers Lane

Rockville, MD 20857-0001

888-INFO-FDA (888-463-6332)

www.fda.gov

The FDA is a public health agency that enforces the Federal Food, Drug, and Cosmetic Act and other laws; promotes health by helping safe and effective products reach the market in a timely manner; and monitors products for continued safety once they are in use. The Web site has information on FDA-regulated products.

Pain

American Academy of Pain Medicine (AAPM)

4700 West Lake

Glenview, IL 60025

847-375-4731

www.painmed.org

The AAPM is the medical specialty society for physicians practicing pain medicine. The academy is involved in education, training, advocacy, and research in pain medicine. The AAPM Web site has links to other sites related to pain and pain medicine and features membership information and links to the academy's publications and products.

American Chronic Pain Association (ACPA)

PO Box 850

Rocklin, CA 95677

916-632-0922

800-533-3231

www.theacpa.org

e-mail: acpa@pacbell.net

The ACPA offers information and support for people with chronic pain and their families. The ACPA also strives to raise awareness among those in the medical profession, policy makers, and the general public about living with chronic pain. The Web site has some free, downloadable information about managing pain, as well as an online store offering videos, manuals, and other materials.

American Pain Foundation

201 N. Charles Street, Suite 710

Baltimore, MD 21201-4111

888-615-PAIN (888-615-7246)

www.painfoundation.org

This independent nonprofit organization provides information, education, and advocacy to people with pain. The foundation's Web site has a pain information library, downloadable publications, and useful links about pain.

American Pain Society

4700 West Lake Avenue

Glenview, IL 60025

847-375-4715

www.ampainsoc.org

e-mail: info@ampainsoc.org

The American Pain Society, a nonprofit membership organization of scientists, clinicians, policy analysts, and others, seeks to advance pain-related research, education, treatment, and professional practice. The Web site provides limited publications on pain, which can either be viewed online or ordered for a fee.

Mental Health

American Association for Marriage and Family Therapy (AAMFT)
112 South Alfred Street
Alexandria, VA 22314
703-838-9808

www.aamft.org

The AAMFT is the professional organization for marriage and family therapists. In addition to resources for professionals, the organization provides the public with referrals to marriage and family therapists. They also provide educational materials on living with illness and other issues related to families and health.

American Counseling Association (ACA)
5999 Stevenson Avenue
Alexandria, VA 22304
800-347-6647
703-823-6862 (TDD)

www.counseling.org

The ACA is a nonprofit professional and educational organization that supports the counseling profession. The Web site has information for students, consumers, and counselors.

American Psychiatric Association (APA)
1000 Wilson Boulevard, Suite 1825
Arlington, VA 22209-3901
888-35-PSYCH

www.psych.org

The 35,000-plus U.S. and international physicians belonging to this medical specialty society work together to provide humane care and effective treatment for anyone with mental disorder, including mental retardation and substance-related disorders. The Web site includes information about the American Psychiatric Association and links to related organizations.

American Psychological Association (APA)
750 First Street NE
Washington, DC 20002-4242
800-374-2721
202-336-6123 (TDD/TTY)

www.apa.org

The American Psychological Association offers referrals to psychologists in local areas and provides information on family issues, parenting, and health. Its Web site has links to state psychological associations that may also provide local referrals.

National Association of Social Workers (NASW)
750 First Street NE, Suite 700
Washington, DC 20002-4241
202-408-8600

www.socialworkers.org

The NASW is the world's largest membership organization of professional social workers. NASW enhances the professional growth and development of its members, creates and maintains professional standards, and advances sound social policies. The Web site has information and links for professionals and the general public. Publications can be ordered online for a fee.

Spiritual

American Association of Pastoral Counselors (AAPC)
9504A Lee Highway
Fairfax, VA 22031-2303
703-352-7725

www.aapc.org

The AAPC offers an online directory of certified pastoral counselors across the country, as well as links to other relevant resources.

Caregivers and Other Support

Air Charity Network (formerly AirLifeLine and Angel FlightAmerica)
4300 Westgrove Drive
Addison, TX 75001
Phone 877-858-7788

www.aircharitynetwork.org

This is a national network of several independent member organizations providing free flights by volunteer pilots, who use their own private planes to transport patients who cannot afford the cost of commercial flights to their medical facility.

American Association of Retired People (AARP)

601 E Street NW
Washington, DC 20049
888-687-2277

www.aarp.org

www.aarppharmacy.com (pharmacy service)

The AARP is a nonprofit membership organization open to anyone age 50 or older. Its member services include information on managed and long-term care, Medicare, and Medicaid. The Web site has information on a pharmacy service that offers discounts on drugs for cancer treatment and pain relief.

National Family Caregivers Association

10400 Connecticut Avenue, Suite 500
Kensington, MD 20895-3944
800-896-3650

www.nfcacares.org

e-mail: info@thefamilycaregiver.org

The NFCA provides education, support, and advocacy for family caregivers. The Web site offers publications and other materials for purchase, as well as some free, downloadable information. There are also links to other Web sites that provide information about specific diseases and disabilities, as well as other health care issues.

The Well Spouse Foundation

63 West Main Street, Suite H
Freehold, NJ 07728
800-838-0879

www.wellspouse.org

e-mail: info@wellspouse.org

Well Spouse is a national nonprofit membership organization that offers support to wives, husbands, and partners of the chronically ill and/or disabled. Support groups meet monthly. The Web site provides information about how to become a member, meeting times and places, activities, conferences, printed material, and links to other relevant organizations.

Other

American Association of Sex Educators, Counselors, and Therapists

PO Box 1960
Ashland, VA 23005-1960
804-752-0026

www.aasect.org

AASECT is a nonprofit, interdisciplinary professional organization that promotes understanding of human sexuality and healthy sexual behavior. In addition to sex educators, sex counselors, and sex therapists, AASECT members include physicians, nurses, social workers, psychologists, allied health professionals, clergy members, lawyers, sociologists, marriage and family planning specialists, and researchers, as well as students in relevant professional disciplines. The Web site offers information for the public and professionals, with links to a variety of related organizations.

Council of State Administrators of Vocational Rehabilitation (CSAVR)

4733 Bethesda Avenue, Suite 330
Bethesda, MD 20814
301-654-8414

www.rehabnetwork.org

CSAVR consists of the chief administrators of the public rehabilitation agencies, which serve individuals with physical and mental disabilities in the Unites States and its territories. The council is the only national organization that advocates for the Public Vocational Rehabilitation Program. Its mission is to maintain and enhance a national program of public vocational rehabilitation services so that individuals with disabilities can achieve employment, economic self-sufficiency, independence, and inclusion and integration into the community.

Appendix C

Reading List

INTRODUCTION

Barrett, Erin, and Jack Mingo. *Doctors Killed George Washington*. Newburyport, MA: Conari Press, 2002.

Chopra, Deepak. *Journey into Healing*. New York: Three Rivers Press, 1994.

Michael, Jan. *Flying Crooked*. Vancouver: Greystone Books, 2005.

Sontag, Susan. *Illness as Metaphor and AIDS and Its Metaphors*. New York: Picador, 2001.

CHAPTER 1

Ansay, A. Manette. *Limbo*. New York: William Morrow, 2001.

Harpham, Wendy Schlessel. *Happiness in a Storm*. New York: W. W. Norton, 2005.

Taylor, Stacy. *Living Well with a Hidden Disability*. With Robert Epstein. Oakland, CA: New Harbinger Publications, 1999.

CHAPTER 2

Frankl, Viktor. *Man's Search for Meaning*. Boston: Beacon Press, 2006.

Jampolsky, Lee. *Healing Together*. Hoboken, NJ: Wiley, 2002.

Jeffers, Susan. *Embracing Uncertainty*. New York: St. Martin's Press, 2003.

Martin L. B. et al. "Prolonged separation delays wound healing in monogamous California mice, *Peromyscus californicus*, but not in polygynous white-footed mice, *P. leucopus*." *Physiology & Behavior* 87 (2006): 837–41.

Mehl-Madrona, L. "Connectivity and healing: some hypotheses about the phenomenon and how to study it." *Advances in Mind Body Medicine* 2 (2005): 3.

Moore, David Leon. "Maier expected to miss games." *USA Today*, August 27, 2001.

Osborn, Claudia L. *Over My Head*. Kansas City: Andrews McMeel Publishing, 1998.

Pratt, Maureen. *Peace in the Storm*. New York: Galilee Books, 2005.

CHAPTER 3

Bridges, William. *The Way of Transition*. Cambridge, MA: De Capo Press, 2001.

Broaddus, Cindi. *A Random Act*. With Kimberly Lohman Suiters. New York: William Morrow, 2005.

Gonzales, Laurence. *Deep Survival*. New York: W. W. Norton, 2003.

Harpham, Wendy Schlessel. *Happiness in a Storm*. New York: W. W. Norton, 2005.

Moore Lappé, Frances, and Jeffrey Perkins. *You Have the Power*. New York: Tarcher, 2004.

CHAPTER 4

Arnold Bennett. *How to Live on 24 hours a Day*. Hyattsville, MD: Shambling Gates Press, 2000.

Domar, Alice, and Henry Dreher. *Self-Nurture*. New York: Penguin, 2000.

Gallagher, Hugh Gregory. "Growing Old with Polio: A Personal Perspective." In *Post-Polio Syndrome*, edited by Lauro S. Halstead and Gunnar Grimby, 215–22. Philadelphia: Hanley and Belfus, 1995.

Gilbert, Daniel. *Stumbling on Happiness*. New York: Alfred A. Knopf, 2006.

Hallowell, Edward M. *Connect*. New York: Pocket Books, 1999.

Heller, Richard and Rachael Heller. *Healthy Selfishness*. Des Moines: Meredith Books, 2006.

Hewitt, Maria, Sheldon Greenfield and Ellen Stovall, eds. *From Cancer Patient to Cancer Survivor*. Washington, DC: National Academies Press, 2006.

Levy, Naomi. *To Begin Again*. New York: Ballantine Books, 1998.

Moore, Thomas. *Dark Nights of the Soul*. New York: Gotham Books, 2004.

Muller, Wayne. *Sabbath*. New York: Bantam Books, 1999.

Page, Susan. *How One of You Can Bring the Two of You Together*. New York: Broadway Books, 1997.

Praver, Frances Cohen. *Crossroads at Midlife*. Westport, CT: Praeger Publishers, 2004.

Rich, Katherine Russell. *The Red Devil*. New York: Three Rivers Press, 1999.

Wolfe, Virginia. "On Being Ill." In *The Moment and Other Essays*. New York: Harcourt Brace & Company, 1948.

CHAPTER 5

Csikszentmihalyi, Mihaly. *Flow: The Psychology of Optimal Experience*. New York: Harper Perennial, 1990.

Emery, C. F. et al. "Exercise accelerates wound healing among healthy older adults: A preliminary investigation." *Journal of Gerontology* 11 (2005): 1432–36.

Miller, B. F., et al. "Coordinated collagen and muscle protein synthesis in human patella tendon and quadriceps muscle after exercise." *Journal of Physiology* 567 (2005): 1021–33.

Valeri, C. R., and M. D. Altschule. *Hypovolemic Anemia of Trauma: The Missing Blood Syndrome*. Boca Raton, FL: Chemical Rubber Company Press, 1981.

CHAPTER 6

Crews, F. T. et al. "Cytokines and alcohol." *Alcoholism: Clinical and Experimental Research* 30 (2006): 720–30.

Degoutte, F. et al. "Food restriction, performance, biochemical, psychological, and endocrine changes in judo athletes." *International Journal of Sports Medicine* 27 (2006): 9–18.

Frieman, A. et al. "Cutaneous effects of smoking." *Journal of Cutaneous Medicine and Surgery* 8 (2004): 415–23.

Prose, Francine. *Gluttony*. New York: Oxford University Press, 2003.

Saper, R. B. et al. "Heavy metal content of ayurvedic herbal medicine products." *Journal of the American Medical Association* 292 (2004): 2868–73.

Willett, Walter. *Eat, Drink, and Be Healthy*. New York: Free Press, 2001.

CHAPTER 7

Christensen, M. "Noise levels in a general surgical ward: a descriptive study." *Journal of Clinical Nursing* 14 (2005): 156–64.

Epstein, Lawrence, and Steven Mardon. *The Harvard Medical School Guide to a Good Night's Sleep*. New York: McGraw-Hill, 2006.

Jones, C. B. et al. "Fatigue and the criminal law." *Industrial Health* 43 (2005): 63–70.

Malik, S. W., and J. Kaplan. "Sleep deprivation." *Primary Care: Clinics in Office Practice* 32 (2005): 475–90.

Parthasarathy, S., and M. J. Tobin. "Sleep in the intensive care unit." *Intensive Care Medicine* 30 (2004): 197–206.

Rogers, N. L. et al. "Neuroimmunologic aspects of sleep and sleep loss." *Seminars in Clinical Neuropsychiatry* 6 (2001): 295–307.

CHAPTER 8

Brallier, Jess M., ed. *Medical Wit & Wisdom*. Philadelphia: Running Press, 1993.

Carroll, L. J., J. D. Cassidy, and P. Côté. "Frequency, timing and course of depressive symptomatology after whiplash." *Spine* 31 (2006): E551–56.

Huth, Edward J., and T. Jock Murray, eds. *Medicine in Quotations*. Philadelphia: American College of Physicians, 2006.

Loeser, John D. et al. *Bonica's Management of Pain*. 3rd ed. Philadelphia: Lippincott, Williams & Wilkins, 2001.

Silver, Julie K. *After Cancer Treatment*. Baltimore: Johns Hopkins University Press, 2006.

Zelman, D. C. et al. "Sleep impairment in patients with painful diabetic peripheral neuropathy." *Clinical Journal of Pain* 22 (2006): 681–85.

CHAPTER 9

Cousins, Norman. *Anatomy of an Illness as Perceived by the Patient*. New York: W. W. Norton, 1979.

Dossey, Larry. *Healing Beyond the Body*. Boston: Shambhala, 2003.

Dreher, Henry. *Mind-Body Unity*. Baltimore: The Johns Hopkins University Press, 2003.

Fleshner, M., and M. L. Laudenslager. "Psychoneuroimmunology: Then and now." *Behavioral and Cognitive Neuroscience Reviews* 3 (2004): 114–30.

Kliger, Benjamin, and Roberta Lee, eds. *Integrative Medicine*. New York: McGraw-Hill, 2004.

Paquette, M. "The mind-body link enters the mainstream." *Perspectives in Psychiatric Care* 40 (2004): 3–4.

Salerno, Steve. *Sham: How the Self-Help Movement Made America Helpless*. New York: Crown Publishers, 2005.

CHAPTER 10

Broadbent, E. et al. "Psychological stress impairs early wound repair following surgery." *Psychosomatic Medicine* 65 (2003): 865–69.

Cohen, Richard. *Blindsided: Lifting a Life Above Illness*. New York: HarperCollins, 2004.

Frank, Arthur W. *At the Will of the Body*. Boston: Mariner Books, 2002.

Hallowell, Edward M. *Worry: Help and Hope for a Common Condition*. New York: Ballantine, 1998.

Helfant, Richard. *Courageous Confrontations*. Boulder, CO: Sentient Publications, 2005.

Holland, Jimmie C., and Sheldon Lewis. *The Human Side of Cancer*. New York: Quill, 2000.

Laurent, C. "Wounds heal more quickly if patients are relieved of stress." *British Medical Journal* 327 (2003): 522.

Marucha, P. T. et al. "Mucosal wound healing is impaired by examination stress." *Psychosomatic Medicine* 60 (1998): 362–65.

Naparstek, Belleruth. *Invisible Heroes*. New York: Bantam Books, 2004.

Silver, Julie. *After Cancer Treatment*. Baltimore: The Johns Hopkins University Press, 2006.

Ubel, Peter. *You're Stronger Than You Think*. New York: McGraw-Hill, 2006.

Westberg, Granger E. *Good Grief*. Minneapolis: Fortress Press, 1997.

CHAPTER 11

Becker, Suzy. *I Had Brain Surgery, What's Your Excuse?* New York: Workman Publishing, 2005.

Brown, S. L. et al. "Providing social support may be more beneficial than receiving it: results from a prospective study of mortality." *Psychological Science* 14 (2003): 320–27.

Campbell, Susan. *Saying What's Real*. Tiburon, CA: H. J. Kramer Books, 2005.

Giles, L. C. et al. "Effect of social networks on 10 year survival in very old Australians: the Australian longitudinal study of aging." *Journal of Epidemiology and Community Health* 59 (2005): 574–79.

Hallowell, Edward M. *Connect*. New York: Pocket Books, 1999.

Harpham, Wendy S. *When a Parent Has Cancer*. New York: HarperCollins, 1997.

Heiss, Gayle. *Finding the Way Home: A Compassionate Approach to Illness*. Fort Bragg, CA: QED Press, 1997.

Hendrix, Harville, and Helen LaKelly Hunt. *Receiving Love*. New York: Atria Books, 2004.

Kiecolt-Glaser, J. K. et al. "Hostile marital interactions, proinflammatory cytokine production, and wound healing." *Archives of General Psychiatry* 62 (2005): 1377–84.

Kraut, R. et al. "Internet paradox: a social technology that reduces social involvement and psychological well-being?" *The American Psychologist* 53 (1998): 1017–31.

Lerner, Harriet. *The Dance of Connection*. New York: Quill, 2002.

Lucas, Geralyn. *Why I Wore Lipstick to My Mastectomy*. New York: St. Martin's Griffin, 2004.

Mehl-Madrona, L. "Connectivity and healing: some hypotheses about the phenomenon and how to study it." *Advances in Mind Body Medicine* 2 (2005): 3.

Ornish, Dean. *Love and Survival*. NewYork: HarperCollins, 1998.

Osborn, Claudia L. *Over My Head*. Kansas City: Andrews McMeel Publishing, 1998.

Page, Susan. *How One of You Can Bring the Two of You Together*. New York: Broadway Books, 1997.

Pratt, Maureen. *Peace in the Storm*. New York: Galilee Books, 2005.

Rauch, Paula K., and Anna C. Muriel. *Raising an Emotionally Healthy Child When a Parent Is Sick*. New York: McGraw-Hill, 2006.

Rodgers, Joni. *Bald in the Land of Big Hair*. New York: HarperCollins, 2001.

Rollin, Betty. *First, You Cry*. New York: HarperCollins Publishers, 2000.

Schlessel Harpham, Wendy. *When a Parent Has Cancer*. New York: HarperCollins, 1997.

Schnipper, Hester Hill. *After Breast Cancer: A Common-Sense Guide to Life After Treatment*. New York: Random House, 2003.

CHAPTER 12

Boudreaux, E. D. et al. "Spiritual role in healing: An alternative way of thinking." *Primary Care* 29 (2002): 439–54.

Carter, Stephen L. "The power of prayer denied." *New York Times*, January 31, 1996.

Dossey, Larry. *Prayer is Good Medicine*. San Francisco: HarperSanFrancisco, 1997.

DuBray, Wynne, ed. *Spirituality and Healing: A Multicultural Perspective*. New York: Writers Club Press, 2001.

Karff, Samuel E. "Healing of body, healing of spirit." *CCAR Journal: A Reform Jewish Quarterly* (2004): 85–95.

Kliewer, S. "Allowing spirituality into the healing process." *Journal of Family Practice* 53 (2004): 616–24.

Koenig, H.G. et al. "Attendance at religious services, interleukin-6, and other biological parameters of immune function in older adults." *International Journal of Psychiatry in Medicine* 27 (1997): 233–50.

Kushner, Harold. *Who Needs God*. New York: Fireside, 1989.

MacNutt, Francis. *The Power to Heal*. Notre Dame, IN: Ave Maria Press, 2004.

Mansfield, C. J., J. Mitchell, and D. E. King. "The doctor as God's mechanic? Beliefs in the Southeastern United States." *Social Science & Medicine* 54 (2002): 399–409.

Marty, Martin E. "Religion and Healing: The Four Expectations." In *Religion and Healing in America*, edited by Linda L. Barnes and Susan S. Sered. New York: Oxford University Press, 2005.

McClelland, D. C. "The effect of motivational arousal through films on salivary immunoglobulin A." *Psychology and Health* 2 (1988): 31–52.

McGrath, Thomas. *Raising Faith-Filled Kids*. Chicago: Loyal Press, 2000.

Pert, Candace. *Everything You Need to Know to Feel Go(o)d*. With Nancy Marriott. Carlsbad, CA: Hay House, 2006.

Polkinghorne, John. *Belief in God in an Age of Science*. New Haven: Yale University Press, 1998.

Qidwai, W., and A. Tayyab. "Patients' views about physicians' spiritual role in medical practice." *Journal of the College of Physicians and Surgeons, Pakistan* 14 (2004): 462–65.

Sayers, Gale. *I Am Third*. With Al Silverman. New York: Viking Press, 1970.

Schuller, Robert A. *Getting Through What You're Going Through*. Corning, CA: Nelson Books, 2006.

Shuman, Joel James, and Keith G. Meador. *Heal Thyself: Spirituality, Medicine, and the Distortion of Christianity*. New York: Oxford University Press, 2003.

CHAPTER 13

Breslau, Karen. "Healing war's wounds." *Newsweek,* September 11, 2006.

Charlton, James, ed. *The Military Quotation Book*. New York: Thomas Dunne Books, 2002.

Klauser, Henriette Anne. *Write It Down, Make It Happen*. New York: Touchstone, 2000.

Klug, Chris and Steve Jackson. *To the Edge and Back: My Story from Organ Transplant Survivor to Olympic Snowboarder*. New York: Carroll & Graff, 2004.

CHAPTER 14

Davis, Nancy. *Lean on Me*. New York: Fireside, 2006.

Edwards, Elizabeth. *Saving Graces: Finding Solace and Strength from Friends and Strangers*. New York: Broadway Books, 2006.

Kaelin, Carolyn. *Living Through Breast Cancer*. New York: McGraw-Hill, 2005.

CHAPTER 15

Murray, W. H. *The Scottish Himalayan Expedition*. London: J. M. Dent & Sons, 1951.

Phillips, Robert H. *Rising to the Challenge: Celebrities and Their Very Personal Health Stories*. Garden City Park, NY: Avery Publishing Group, 1990.

Index